Strength Fitness

Physiological Principles
and
Training Techniques

Third Edition

Strength Fitness

Physiological Principles and Training Techniques

Third Edition

Wayne Westcott
South Shore YMCA

WCB Wm. C. Brown Publishers

Book Team

Editor *Chris Rogers*
Developmental Editor *Cindy Kuhrasch*
Production Coordinator *Carla D. Arnold*

WCB **Wm. C. Brown Publishers**

President *G. Franklin Lewis*
Vice President, Publisher *George Wm. Bergquist*
Vice President, Publisher *Thomas E. Doran*
Vice President, Operations and Production *Beverly Kolz*
National Sales Manager *Virginia S. Moffat*
Advertising Manager *Ann M. Knepper*
Editor in Chief *Edward G. Jaffe*
Production Editorial Manager *Colleen A. Yonda*
Production Editorial Manager *Julie A. Kennedy*
Publishing Services Manager *Karen J. Slaght*
Manager of Visuals and Design *Faye M. Schilling*

Cover photo by Mike Ryan and Kevin Forti

Cover design by John R. Rokusek

Copyright © 1987, 1983 by Allyn and Bacon, Inc.

Copyright © 1989, 1991 by Wm. C. Brown Publishers. All rights
reserved

Library of Congress Catalog Card Number: 89-86045

ISBN 0-697-10629-2

Printed in the United States of America by Wm. C. Brown Publishers,
2460 Kerper Boulevard, Dubuque, IA 52001

10 9 8 7 6 5 4 3 2

To my wife and our parents,
for their prayers and encouragement

Contents

Preface

When asked about strength training, most people think about bodybuilders, weightlifters, or football players. They typically view strength training as important to these individuals but as rather irrelevant to themselves. Although there has been considerable progress since the first edition of *Strength Fitness* was published in 1983, many adults still do not realize the significant physical benefits they can enjoy through sensible strength training. In addition, they are often unaware how little time is necessary to obtain relatively high levels of muscular conditioning.

This is unfortunate because with respect to strength training, what people don't know can hurt them. For example, most men and women have no idea that unless they perform regular strength exercise they lose approximately five pounds of muscle every ten years. Neither do they understand that this steady loss of muscle is largely responsible for lowering their metabolic rate by 5 percent every decade. They seldom consider the fact that 80 percent of low back problems are muscular in nature. With almost four out of five Americans experiencing some degree of low back discomfort, this alone should be sufficient motivation to participate in a strength fitness program.

But there are many other reasons that every person should pursue sensible strength training. Muscles function as our shock absorbers, our engines, and our chassis. That is, well-conditioned muscles reduce our risk of injury, increase our physical capacity, and enhance our personal appearance.

While a reasonable amount of effort and commitment are necessary to experience muscular fitness, strength training need not be a time-consuming activity. Generally speaking, twenty to thirty minutes of regular and properly performed strength exercise are sufficient for achieving significant strength gains in all of the major muscle groups. Of course, safe, effective, and efficient training sessions are dependent upon sound physiological principles and sensible training techniques.

Because application is just as important as knowledge, this edition of *Strength Fitness* includes a comprehensive chapter on program design and management, with special emphasis on staff instruction, member orientation, and personal motivation. Like the previous editions, it also presents updated information on strength physiology, performance factors, training recommendations, and exercise techniques.

The intent of this book is to help fitness professionals (teachers, coaches, and instructors) develop a better understanding of strength training in order to help others attain higher levels of strength fitness. If this objective is to be realized, it will certainly be through the collective efforts of educators and practitioners alike.

The author acknowledges Ellington Darden, Ted Lambrinides, Joseph Martino, Mary Moore, and Ralph Yohe for their help and encouragement in producing this book. Special appreciation is extended to Wes Emmert, Certified Strength and Conditioning Coach at Boston College, for his invaluable assistance with both the text and photographs in chapter 7. The author is also grateful to Dianne Cirino, Wes Emmert, Chris Gildea, Charles Hardesty, BethAnne Strenge, and Claudia Westcott for modeling the Strength Training Exercises throughout chapters 6 and 7. In addition, the precise figures by Leslie Willis, and the excellent photographs by Mike Ryan and Kevin Forti are much appreciated. The following reviewers also deserve acknowledgment: Lorraine R. Brilla, Western Washington University; Larry A. Good, Southern Illinois University; Robert Haslam, Bridgewater State College; Martin W. Johnson, Mayville State University; William J. Meadors, Western Kentucky University; Dick Prentice, Delta College; Nancy Rich, Miami University; and Donna Terbizan, North Dakota State University. Finally, sincere thanks to my Administrative Assistant, Susan Ramsden, for typing the manuscript for this text, and to my wife, Claudia, for directing a model strength fitness facility.

One

Strength Training Benefits

Strength training is often referred to as progressive resistance exercise. In simplest terms, strength training is a systematic means of adding resistance to various exercise movements. Of course, in order to handle greater resistance positive adaptations must take place within the musculoskeletal system.

The basic beneficial changes that result from strength training are increased contractile strength in muscles and increased tensile strength in tendons, ligaments, and bones (Zuckerman and Stull 1969; Mathews and Fox 1976; Nutter 1986; Fleck and Kraemer 1987).

Strength training enhances muscle contractile strength in two ways. First, it stimulates neural adaptations resulting in better muscle fiber recruitment (Ikai and Fukunaga 1970; Moritani and DeVries 1979; Hakkinen and Komi 1983). Second, it produces more actin and myosin protein filaments resulting in larger and stronger muscle fibers (Gordon 1967; MacDougall et al. 1979).

Although strength training is essential for developing larger and stronger muscles, very few individuals possess the genetic potential to become competitive bodybuilders or weightlifters. Nonetheless, sensible strength training can benefit just about everyone with regard to physical capacity, metabolic function, athletic power, injury prevention, and physical appearance.

Physical Capacity

Physical capacity is a rather complex concept that includes muscular strength and cardiovascular endurance. Both components are important, and both can be improved through proper training. For example, jogging is an excellent means for enhancing cardiovascular endurance, and strength training is an excellent means for increasing muscular strength.

While the heart functions as the fuel pump of the body, the muscles are analogous to the engine of an automobile. It is the muscles where combustion takes place, where energy is released, where movement originates, and where power is produced. Regular strength training increases the muscles' ability to perform work, particularly high-intensity exercise against relatively heavy resistance.

As presented in chapter 4, previously untrained men may experience a 40 percent improvement in muscle performance after one month of strength training. Such improvements, the result of better muscle fiber recruitment and larger muscle fibers, are easily observable and highly motivating to the participants.

It is important to understand that every physical activity requires a certain percentage of one's maximum physical capacity. Because muscle strength and muscle endurance are closely related, more muscle strength results in more muscle endurance with a given resistance (see chapter 4). That is, strength training enables one to produce more work at a particular exercise level and to perform previously difficult tasks with much less effort.

Strong muscles enhance our physical capacity, and our physical capacity has a major influence on our daily lifestyle.

Metabolic Function

Because muscles are the engines of the body, strength training can have a significant influence on our metabolic function. Strength exercise is a vigorous, calorie burning activity (Wilmore et al. 1978). During a high-intensity strength training session, one's heart rate, blood pressure, and energy metabolism increase considerably (see chapter 4).

Of course, this temporary elevation in energy consumption is experienced during other large muscle activities such as running, cycling, and swimming. Endurance training burns more calories than strength training (Hempel and Wells 1985), but after endurance exercise one's metabolism normally returns to resting level within forty minutes (Clark 1985).

Strength training is different in that it influences one's resting metabolism as well as one's exercise metabolism. This is due to the fact that strength training typically increases the amount of muscle tissue, and muscle tissue requires a constant supply of energy to sustain cellular functions. The more muscle one develops, the more energy is necessary twenty-four hours a day for protein synthesis and tissue maintenance. Even during sleep, the skeletal muscles contribute about 25 percent of one's total calorie utilization (Lamb 1985).

After age twenty, men and women who do not perform muscle strengthening activity lose approximately 0.5 pounds of muscle every year simply through lack of use (Forbes 1976). This reduction in muscle tissue may be largely responsible for the decline in metabolic rate that seems to accompany the aging process. Research by Keyes et al. (1973) showed that men experienced a 0.5 percent reduction in metabolic rate every year between twenty-two and fifty years of age. It is therefore advisable for adults to perform regular strength exercise to maintain a desirable level of muscle mass and metabolic function.

Strength exercise is unique in that it has a double effect on energy utilization. First, strength training produces a large increase in metabolic rate during the workout. Second, strength training produces more muscle tissue, thereby establishing a higher resting metabolism and burning calories at a faster rate all day long.

For these reasons, strength training is helpful in reducing body fat. In one study (Westcott 1987b), seventy-two adults followed the same dietary guidelines and spent the same amount of time in an exercise program (thirty minutes a day, three days a week). Twenty-two subjects spent all thirty minutes performing endurance activity. The other fifty participants divided each workout into fifteen minutes of endurance exercise and fifteen minutes of strength exercise. After eight weeks, the subjects who did endurance training only lost 3.0 pounds of fat and 0.5 pounds of muscle. The subjects who performed both strength and endurance exercise lost 10.0 pounds of fat and gained 2.0 pounds of muscle. In the author's opinion, the better results obtained by strength trained subjects were partly due to their increased muscle mass and metabolic rate.

Athletic Power

Successful sports performance is largely dependent upon the athlete's ability to produce power. Almost every athletic event has a power component. Power is most evident in activities such as putting a shot, punting a football, hitting a baseball, dunking a basketball, and sprinting one hundred yards. But power is also involved in running a five-mile race. Assuming similar bodyweights, all of the racers perform about the same amount of work. The winner, however, performs the work in the least amount of time and therefore exhibits the most power (power = work/time).

In simplest terms, power is the combination of two factors, movement speed and muscle force. Generally speaking, increasing one's movement speed and muscle force will result in greater performance power. Movement speed may be improved through high-quality skill training, and muscle force may be improved through high-intensity strength training. Although both power components are important for optimal athletic performance, the author prefers to practice each component separately: skill training to develop movement speed and strength training to develop muscle force.

Consider how strength training may benefit a technical athletic skill such as driving a golf ball. The golfer may gain distance by swinging the club faster, but at some point control may be lost and accuracy may be sacrificed. The golfer may also gain distance by developing greater muscle force through a well-designed strength training program. In this manner, the golfer may increase his driving distance and maintain his striking accuracy because he does not have to alter his normal swing.

It should be noted that increased muscle strength does not necessarily hinder movement speed or joint flexibility (Sewall and Micheli 1986; Finamore 1989). In fact, proper strength training may enhance joint flexibility by alternately stressing and stretching opposing muscle groups through a full range of movement.

Several years ago, athletes were advised to avoid strength training altogether. More recently, coaches encouraged athletes to perform specific strength exercises for the muscles most involved in their event. Although this was a step in the right direction, it often resulted in muscle imbalance and led to overuse injuries. Today, most professional and collegiate athletic teams employ strength coaches to design balanced strength training programs that develop strong athletes and reduce the risk of injury. Proper strength training is undoubtedly a major contributing factor to the outstanding athletic performances of our day.

Injury Prevention

The body, like an automobile, needs shock absorbers to prevent serious problems due to potentially damaging external forces. It also requires balancing agents to prevent serious problems from potentially destructive internal forces. A well-conditioned and well-balanced muscular system serves both of these functions.

One reason an active individual should perform strength training is to reduce the risk of injuries. Since World War II, progressive resistance exercise has been the preferred method of injury rehabilitation. It is now understood that proper strength training may be equally useful as a means of injury prevention (Cahill and Griffith 1978; Hejna et al. 1982). The heavy emphasis on strength training by football coaches undoubtedly contributed to the 44 percent reduction of fatal injuries in this sport from 1975 to 1981 (Mueller and Blyth 1982).

A strong musculoskeletal system offers some protection against injuries, but a balanced musculoskeletal system is even more effective. While some athletic injuries are caused by collisions, most are the result of overtraining one muscle group and undertraining its counterpart. For example, distance runners frequently encounter injuries to the knee joint. Part of the problem is that distance running overstresses the posterior leg muscles and understresses the anterior leg muscles. This creates a front-to-back muscle imbalance that reduces the integrity of the knee joint and predisposes it to injury.

Although solutions are seldom simple, a first step to improve this situation is balanced strength training for all of the leg muscles. When all of the leg muscles are strong, there is considerably less chance of one muscle group overpowering another and causing an imbalance injury.

Of course, it is also advisable for distance runners to strengthen their midsection and upper body muscles. Repetitive running places much stress on the lower back, so a strong midsection (front, back, and sides) is helpful for preventing low back injuries. Because the upper body muscles are powerfully involved in the latter stages of a race, they should also be strengthened in a balanced manner.

Running is not unique. Every athletic event involves some muscle groups more than others, and promotes a degree of muscle imbalance. Therefore, athletes should consider strength training for purposes of maintaining muscle balance and preventing overuse injuries, as well as for improving performance.

Athletes are not the only people who encounter muscle imbalance injuries. Business persons who sit all day and drivers who ride all day place more stress on their low back muscles than their abdominal muscles. As a result, many sedentary men and women experience low back pain. Because 80 percent of low back problems are muscular in nature, strength training may be beneficial from a preventive perspective (Melleby 1982).

It is emphasized that proper strength training can improve muscle balance and reduce the risk of injury. Conversely, improper strength training can be the cause of injury (Finamore 1989). Chapter 5 presents important recommendations for designing safe and effective strength training programs.

Physical Appearance

Continuing the automobile analogy, the muscles are similar to the chassis of a car. That is, the muscles of the body are largely responsible for our physical appearance. In fact, the reason many people begin a strength training program is to look better.

Looking fit is largely a matter of muscle conditioning. Basically, strength exercise stimulates muscle fibers to increase in size and strength, thereby enhancing muscle tone and firmness.

Consider the thousands of men and women who have participated in strength training programs during the past decade. Most have experienced favorable improvements in muscle size, muscle strength, muscle tone, and physical appearance, but few have developed large muscles. This may explain why strength training is one of the most popular physical activities among adults.

Take a typical young woman who weighs 130 pounds and is 26 percent body fat (Westcott 1988d). In terms of body composition, bones account for about 14 pounds, organs and skin account for about 34 pounds, fat accounts for about 34 pounds, and muscle contributes about 48 pounds. If she lost 4 pounds of fat and gained 4 pounds of muscle, she would still weigh 130 pounds but be only 23 percent body fat. Although she could lose 4 pounds of fat through diet and endurance exercise, the only way she could gain 4 pounds of muscle is through regular and progressive strength training. And it is the 4 pounds of additional muscle that enhance her muscle strength, muscle tone, and physical appearance.

Strength training is somewhat unique in that the physical changes are readily apparent to the exerciser and to others. Improvements in body composition are usually noticeable after four to eight weeks of training, and these visible reinforcers provide excellent motivation to continue one's exercise program.

Strength Potential

Contrary to advertisements in popular muscle magazines, few persons who practice strength training will develop championship physiques, because the capacity to attain unusual muscle size is largely determined by genetic factors. However, almost everyone has the potential to look better, feel better, and function better as a result of intelligent strength training.

There are three keys to sensible strength training. These are: (1) safety, (2) effectiveness, and (3) efficiency. The first criterion is safety. Regardless of how well a program may appear to work, if it presents a high risk of injury it should be discontinued. For example, explosive weightlifting movements that place excessive stress on muscles, joints, and connective tissue should be avoided whenever possible. Instead, strength training exercises should be performed with reasonable resistance and controlled movement speeds (see chapter 5).

Although many different conditioning programs produce strength improvement, some are more effective than others. Consider calisthenics such as traditional push-ups and sit-ups. Because these bodyweight exercises do not involve progressive resistance, they do not promote a high rate of strength development (see chapter

5). Better results are obtained by isolating individual muscle groups and progressively increasing the exercise resistance.

Because many people have limited time for physical conditioning, training efficiency is often an important consideration. For example, if one set of exercise produces the same degree of strength development as three sets of exercise, this may be a preferred means of training for busy people (see chapter 4).

The following chapters provide detailed information to help the reader understand and implement these basic strength training concepts. Recommendations for exercise selection, exercise frequency, exercise sets, exercise repetitions, exercise speed, exercise time, and exercise order are presented in light of recent research findings, along with practical advice on designing a personal strength training program.

Strength training is an excellent activity for people who value physical fitness and personal appearance. As illustrated in figures 1.1 and 1.2, the human body consists of several muscle groups, all of which have specific roles in movement mechanics. The purpose of this book is to challenge the reader to train these muscle groups sensibly and to attain a satisfying level of strength fitness.

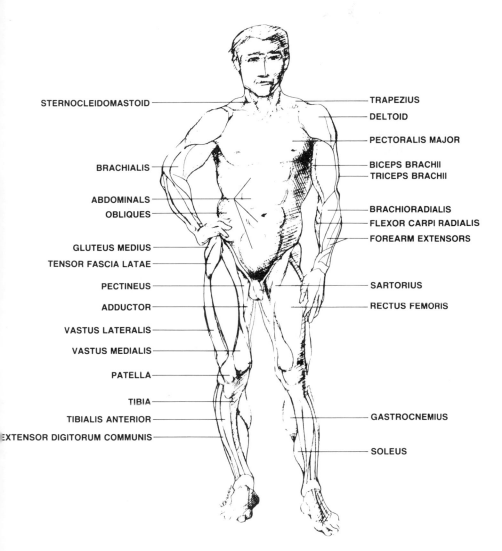

STERNOCLEIDOMASTOID

TRAPEZIUS

DELTOID

PECTORALIS MAJOR

BRACHIALIS

BICEPS BRACHII
TRICEPS BRACHII

ABDOMINALS
OBLIQUES

BRACHIORADIALIS
FLEXOR CARPI RADIALIS
FOREARM EXTENSORS

GLUTEUS MEDIUS
TENSOR FASCIA LATAE

PECTINEUS

SARTORIUS

ADDUCTOR

RECTUS FEMORIS

VASTUS LATERALIS

VASTUS MEDIALIS

PATELLA

TIBIA

TIBIALIS ANTERIOR

GASTROCNEMIUS

EXTENSOR DIGITORUM COMMUNIS

SOLEUS

Figure 1.1 Muscles of the body: front

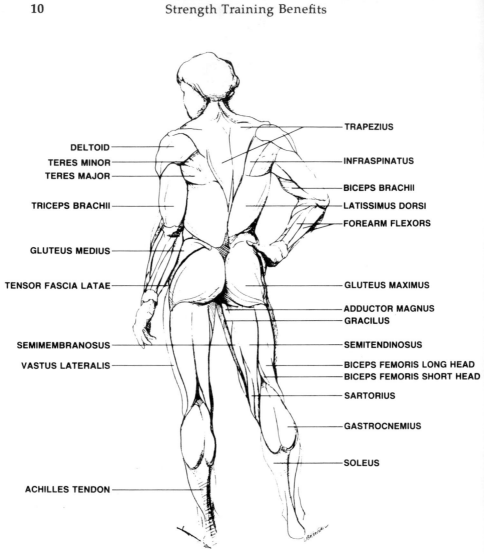

Figure 1.2 Muscles of the body: back

Two

Strength Training Physiology and Kinesiology

In simplest terms, strength training provides a stimulus for muscle growth. Specifically, muscles respond to progressive resistance exercise by developing more actin and myosin protein filaments. The increase in contractile proteins produces larger and stronger muscles that have greater energy requirements.

Muscle Structure

Muscle structure begins with two basic components, thick protein strands called myosin filaments and thin protein strands known as actin filaments. Small projections called cross-bridges extend from the myosin filaments enabling connections with the surrounding actin filaments during muscle contraction. Figure 2.1 illustrates schematically the way these filaments are arranged in a functional contractile unit known as a sarcomere.

Adjacent sarcomeres form myofibrils, which are the principal threads running throughout the muscles. Groups of myofibrils are bound together by a membrane called sarcolemma to form individual muscle fibers. In turn, muscle fibers are bound together by a sheath called perimysium into bundles of fibers known as fasciculi. These bundles of fibers are enclosed by connective tissue called epimysium and function together as a muscle, such as the deltoids. The structural and functional components of skeletal muscle are shown in figure 2.2.

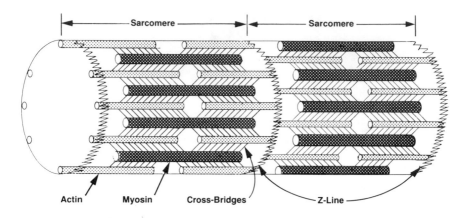

Figure 2.1 The smallest functional unit of muscle contraction, the sarcomere, consists of thin actin filaments, thick myosin filaments, and tiny cross-bridges that serve as coupling agents between the myosin proteins and the surrounding actin proteins

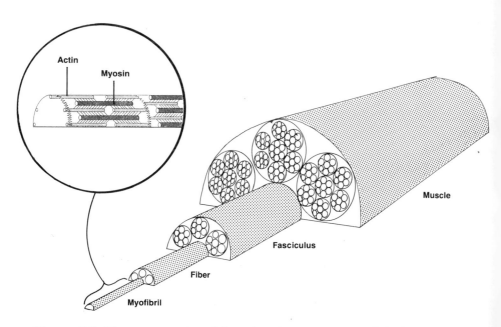

Figure 2.2 The structural and functional components of skeletal muscle

Muscle Physiology

Huxley (1969) proposed that muscles contract when the thick myosin protein filaments pull the thin actin protein filaments toward each other. This is referred to as the sliding filament theory of muscle contraction.

The energy necessary for muscle contraction is obtained from a rapid series of events beginning with nervous stimulation to the muscle cell. Upon receiving the nerve impulse, calcium ions are released from the sarcoplasmic reticulum that surrounds the muscle fiber. The calcium ions attach to two proteins, troponin and tropomyosin, that normally prevent contact between the actin and myosin filaments. With troponin and tropomyosin bound to the calcium ions, myosin proteins function enzymatically to split adenosine triphosphate (ATP) into adenosine diphosphate (ADP), free phosphate (Pi) and energy. The ATP-splitting activity appears to take place at the cross-bridges, providing energy for the actin-myosin linkage and pulling action that is responsible for muscle contraction. Actually, the cross-bridges attach, release and reattach in a series of ratchetlike movements to pull the actin filaments toward the center of the myosin filaments (see figure 2.3).

Upon cessation of the nervous stimulation, the calcium ions are collected into the sarcoplasmic reticulum. This permits troponin and tropomyosin proteins to perform their normal function of preventing contact between the actin and myosin filaments. As a result, the enzymatic activity of the myosin proteins ceases, ATP molecules are not split, energy is not released, cross-linkages do not occur, and the muscle fiber relaxes.

Muscle Contraction

When a muscle is activated, it produces tension and attempts to shorten. That is, it tends to pull its attachments closer together. It should be understood, however, that muscle contraction actually means muscle tension and does not necessarily imply a change in muscle length. A contracting muscle may actually shorten, lengthen, or remain the same size.

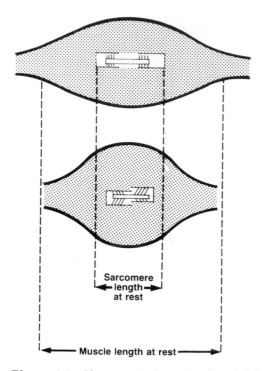

Figure 2.3 Changes in length of individual sarcomeres and entire muscle during concentric muscle contraction

Concentric contraction.   When a barbell is pressed from one's chest during the bench press exercise, the pectoralis major, anterior deltoid, and triceps muscles exert force, shorten, and overcome the weightload. Whenever a muscle exerts force, shortens, and overcomes a resistance, it is said to contract concentrically. Concentric contractions are essential for overcoming the force of gravity and for enabling the exerciser to perform lifting movements.

Eccentric contraction.   When a barbell is lowered to one's chest during the bench press exercise, the pectoralis major, anterior deltoid, and triceps muscles exert force, lengthen, and are overcome by the weightload. Whenever a muscle exerts force, lengthens, and is overcome by a resistance, it is said to contract eccentrically. Note that if these muscles did not exert force during the lowering phase of the bench press exercise, the bar would drop onto the chest with the full force of gravity and cause considerable harm to the lifter. Eccentric contractions are, therefore, important for attenuating the force of gravity and for enabling the exerciser to perform safe, controlled lowering movements.

Isometric contraction.   If a barbell is momentarily held six inches above the chest during the bench press exercise, the pectoralis major, anterior deltoid, and triceps muscles exert force, but do not change in length. They neither overcome the weightload nor are they overcome by the weightload. When a muscle exerts force, but does not change in length, it is said to contract isometrically. In other words, the force exerted by the muscle is equal to the force exerted by the resistance, and no movement occurs. Isometric contractions are important for stabilizing movements and for maintaining given joint positions.

Isotonic Exercise

When lifting or lowering a barbell, the amount of resistive force selected largely determines the amount of muscle force produced. However, due to leverage changes, the effective muscle force varies throughout the movement range. Training performed with a fixed resistance is referred to as isotonic exercise.

Variable Resistance Exercise

Some strength training machines incorporate variable resistance in an attempt to accommodate leverage changes. Through levers, cams, or other designs, the resistive force is decreased or increased in accordance with the effective muscle force. That is, the machines provide more resistance where the effective muscle force is higher and less resistance where the effective muscle force is lower.

Isokinetic Exercise

Other strength training equipment provides accommodating resistance in a different manner. Isokinetic exercise equipment maintains a constant movement speed and varies the resistive force in accordance with the applied muscle force. In other words, more muscle force results in more resistive force and less muscle force results in less resistive force, but the movement speed remains the same. Although most isokinetic machines use only concentric movements, isokinetic exercise can involve both concentric muscle contractions and eccentric muscle contractions.

Prime Mover Muscles

In any given joint action, the muscle that is principally responsible for controlling the movement is termed the prime mover muscle. The prime mover muscle may contract concentrically to lift a weight or contract eccentrically to lower a weight.

As an example, the biceps muscles are principally responsible for elbow flexion movements. Therefore, they are the prime mover muscles for barbell curls (see chapter 7). Many exercises involve more than one prime mover muscle group. Pull-ups, for example, require both shoulder extension and elbow flexion. In this case, the latissimus dorsi, upper back, and posterior deltoid muscles principally responsible for shoulder extension and the biceps muscles principally responsible for elbow flexion are the prime mover groups (see chapter 7).

Antagonistic Muscles

The muscle that produces the opposite joint action to that of the prime mover is called the antagonist. Because they extend the elbow, the triceps muscles are the antagonists of the biceps muscles. On the other hand, the triceps are the prime mover muscles for elbow extension exercises such as triceps extensions (see chapter 7). For smooth elbow flexion, the triceps (antagonists) must relax and lengthen as the biceps (prime movers) contract and shorten. Conversely, for smooth elbow extension, the biceps (antagonists) must relax and lengthen as the triceps (prime movers) contract and shorten.

Stabilizer Muscles

For the desired movements to occur in certain joints, other joints must be stabilized. For example, when performing strict barbell curls, the torso must remain erect and the upper arms must be held against the sides. The first stabilization is accomplished by isometric contraction of the low back muscles. The second stabilization is accomplished by isometric contraction of the pectoralis major and latissimus dorsi muscles.

A similar situation occurs when performing strict push-ups. The midsection muscles must contract isometrically to maintain the body in a straight and stable position. The muscles that perform this stabilizing function are referred to as stabilizer or synergist muscles, because their contraction facilitates the desired action from the prime mover muscles.

Force Production

A muscle contracts when energy (ATP) is released, cross-linkages occur between the actin and myosin filaments, and both ends of the sarcomere are pulled toward the center. This is the mechanism by which muscle force is produced.

Motor Unit

Muscle contraction is regulated by the motor unit. A motor unit is made up of a single motor neuron and all the muscle fibers that receive stimulation from that nerve (see figure 2.4). In large muscles, such as the rectus femoris, a single motor neuron may innervate several hundred muscle fibers. In smaller muscles that produce precise movements, such as the muscles that move the eyes, each motor neuron innervates only a few muscle fibers.

Motor unit recruitment is the key to smooth, forceful, and sustained muscle contraction. Because the muscle fibers in a given motor unit are distributed throughout the muscle, only a few motor units need to be activated for coordinated muscle contraction. This arrangement allows individual motor units to alternately fire and rest when work is performed at submaximal strength levels.

Force Regulation

Because muscles are required to exert varying degrees of force (e.g., placing a light bulb in an overhead socket versus pressing a ninety-pound barbell), some type of regulatory system is essential. There are two factors that affect the strength of a muscle contraction. These are the frequency of nerve impulses and the number of motor units activated. Fine adjustments in muscle tension are produced by changes in the frequency of nerve impulses to the muscle fibers. As the frequency of nerve impulses increases, the strength of contraction increases; and as the frequency of nerve impulses decreases, the strength of contraction decreases. Gross variations in muscle tension

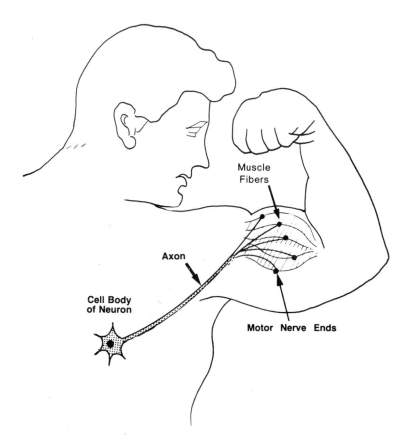

Figure 2.4 The motor unit consists of a single motor nerve and all of the muscle fibers that it innervates

are dependent upon the number of motor units activated by the central nervous system. The more units required, the stronger the contraction and vice versa. Under normal circumstances, different motor units fire independently. When maximum strength is required, nervous impulses may arrive more synchronously to enable the muscle fibers to produce maximum tension.

Force Assessment

According to Jones et al. (1988), muscle force is most accurately measured during a maximum isometric contraction, because muscle movement (concentric and eccentric) involves internal frictional forces. They found that in a fresh muscle, slow concentric contractions underestimate muscle force production by about 17 percent, because internal friction subtracts this amount from the muscle's actual force output. Conversely, they found that slow eccentric contractions overestimate muscle force production by about 17 percent, because internal friction adds this amount to the muscle's actual force output.

For example, Joe produces a maximum isometric contraction of 120 pounds, a maximum concentric contraction (twenty-five degrees/second) of 100 pounds and a maximum eccentric contraction (twenty-five degrees/second) of 140 pounds. His actual muscle force is 120 pounds, with internal friction responsible for both the lower concentric output and the higher eccentric output.

Fiber Types

Although the strength of contraction in skeletal muscles is primarily regulated by the central nervous system, the individual motor units possess different contractile capacities, generally referred to as fast-twitch characteristics or slow-twitch characteristics.

Slow-twitch muscle fibers bear the major burden in activities that require submaximum force production. These fibers are better suited for aerobic energy utilization because they contain more mitochondria, more endurance enzymes, more blood capillaries, and more intramuscular triglyceride stores. They are therefore well-designed for long-term exercise that primarily utilizes oxygen for energy production. Because slow-twitch fibers can produce low-force contractions for relatively long periods of time, these are the dominant muscle fibers among endurance athletes such as marathon runners.

Fast-twitch muscle fibers bear the major burden in activities that require maximum force production. MacDougall (1985a) has reported larger cross-sectional areas, more contractile proteins, and greater training-induced hypertrophy in fast-twitch muscle fibers. These fibers are better suited for anaerobic energy utilization because they have more myosin ATPase activity, more glycolytic enzyme activity, and more intramuscular phosphate stores. They are therefore well-designed for short-term exercise that principally depends upon phosphate breakdown for energy production. Because fast-twitch fibers can produce high-force contractions for relatively short periods of time, these are the dominant muscle fibers among power athletes such as sprinters and jumpers.

Research (Lesmes et al. 1983) indicates that both fast-twitch motor units and slow-twitch motor units are recruited for maximum force production. When submaximum efforts are required, slow-twitch motor units are activated first, followed by fast-twitch motor units if necessary. It is unlikely that one can change the proportion of slow-twitch and fast-twitch muscle fibers through strength training (Dons et al. 1979; Costill et al. 1979; MacDougall et al. 1982).

Fiber Arrangement

Another factor that influences the strength of contraction is the muscle fiber arrangement. There are basically two types of fiber patterns, fusiform and penniform. Fusiform muscles have long fibers that run parallel to the line of pull. Muscles of this type produce less force but have a large range of movement. The biceps femoris muscle of the hamstrings group is fusiform. Penniform muscles have short fibers that run diagonally to the line of pull. Penniform muscles, therefore, produce greater force but have a smaller range of movement. Figure 2.5 presents schematic drawings of a fusiform muscle

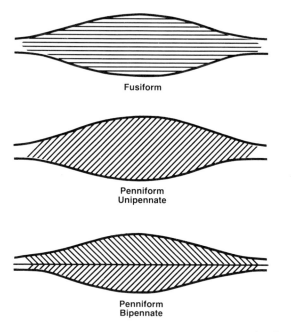

Fusiform

Penniform
Unipennate

Penniform
Bipennate

Figure 2.5 Schematic representations of a fusiform muscle, a unipennate muscle, and a bipennate muscle

and two types of penniform muscles, penniform unipennate and the stronger penniform bipennate. The semitendinosus muscle of the hamstrings group is penniform unipennate, and the rectus femoris muscle of the quadriceps is penniform bipennate.

Muscle Relaxation

The natural state of skeletal muscle is called relaxation. It is recalled that skeletal muscle contracts only upon nervous stimulation to do so. In the absence of such stimulation, the contractile mechanism is inactive, myosin cross-bridges do not connect with actin filaments, and muscle tension is not developed.

An important aspect of muscle relaxation is the ability of an antagonist muscle to relax when a prime mover muscle contracts. This process is known as reciprocal inhibition and is essential for coordinated movements. At the same time that the prime mover muscle is stimulated to contract and shorten, the antagonist muscle is cued to relax and lengthen. Actually, the degree of tension in each of the opposing muscle groups (prime movers and antagonists) is precisely regulated by the nervous system to enable smooth movements with varying degrees of speed and force.

Muscle Protection

The body is equipped with built-in mechanisms to prevent tissue damage as a result of too much muscle tension or too much muscle stretch. Golgi tendon organs, located within the muscle tendons, respond to excessive stress by inhibiting muscle contraction, thereby decreasing potentially dangerous levels of muscle tension.

Muscle spindles, located within the muscles, are sensitive to muscle stretch. Whenever a muscle is stretched too far or too quickly, the muscle spindles trigger a reflex action that causes the muscle to contract, thereby reducing the risk of injury.

Muscle Fatigue

Although the exact mechanisms responsible for muscle fatigue are not fully understood, potential fatigue sites include the central nervous system, the motor nerve, the neuromuscular junction, and the contractile mechanism. More specifically, as a muscle continues to contract forcefully the anaerobic energy sources become temporarily depleted. At the same time, anaerobic waste products such as lactic acid accumulate in the muscle. This increases tissue acidity, which adversely affects contractile ability. In addition, chemical changes at the neuromuscular junctions may prevent further muscle contraction (Lamb 1978).

Muscle fatigue may be experienced in many degrees, up to the point of temporary muscle failure. At temporary muscle failure the muscle is no longer able to contract concentrically and is overcome by the resistance. After a few seconds of recovery the muscle's contractile ability is partially restored, and after two minutes the anaerobic energy sources are largely replaced.

The immediate effect of exercising to muscle failure is varying degrees of discomfort, including muscle tightness and a localized burning sensation. Although this temporary muscle discomfort passes quickly, delayed onset muscle soreness may occur one or two days after the exercise session.

According to MacDougall (1985b), lifting and lowering heavy weights may result in damage to muscle and connective tissue that requires considerable time for repair and rebuilding. Research (Friden et al. 1983; Byrnes and Clarkson 1986) indicates that eccentric contractions cause greater muscle microtrauma (microscopic tissue damage) and are therefore more likely to produce delayed onset muscle soreness.

Musculoskeletal Structure and Function

The function of skeletal muscle is to produce tension that is typically translated into movement. Muscles are attached to bones by connective tissue called tendons, which are actually extensions of the perimysium and epimysium. As illustrated in figure 2.6, contraction of a skeletal muscle generally moves one bone through a range of degrees toward another bone. Generally speaking, the bone that remains stationary is considered the muscle origin and the bone that moves is considered the muscle insertion.

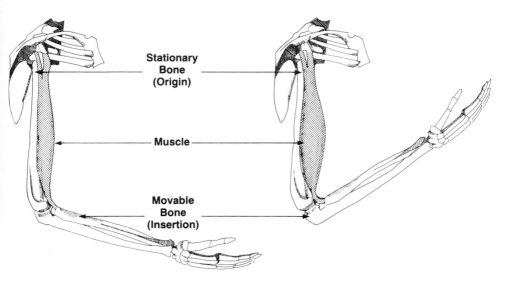

Figure 2.6 Contraction of a muscle resulting in the movement of one bone toward another. The stationary bone is referred to as the muscle origin, and the movable bone as the muscle insertion.

Joint Movements

The focus of this book is movement about the major joints of the human body. More specifically, exercises that, when properly applied, can increase the muscular force of the following joint movements will be presented. The joint movements are illustrated schematically in figure 2.7.

Elbow Flexion: Decreasing the angle between the arm and the forearm.

Elbow Extension: Increasing the angle between the arm and the forearm.

Knee Flexion: Decreasing the angle between the thigh and the leg.

Knee Extension: Increasing the angle between the thigh and the leg.

Shoulder Adduction: Decreasing the angle between the arm and the side (downward-sideward movement).

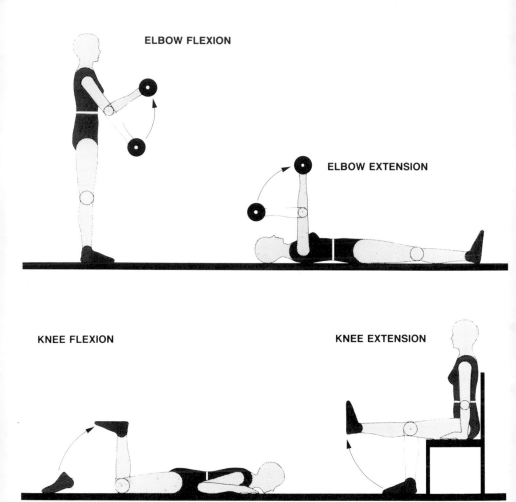

Figure 2.7 Schematic illustrations of joint movements

Shoulder Abduction: Increasing the angle between the arm and the side (upward-sideward movement).

Shoulder Flexion: Increasing the angle between the arm and the chest (upward-forward movement).

Shoulder Extension: Decreasing the angle between the arm and the chest (downward-backward movement).

SHOULDER ADDUCTION   SHOULDER ABDUCTION

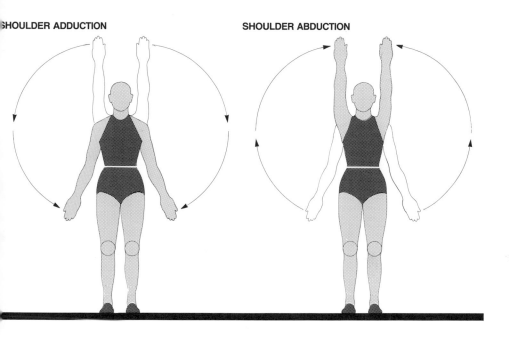

SHOULDER FLEXION   SHOULDER EXTENSION

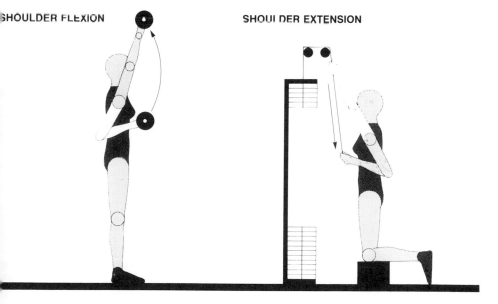

Figure 2.7 *(continued)*

SHOULDER HORIZONTAL FLEXION

SHOULDER HORIZONTAL EXTENSION

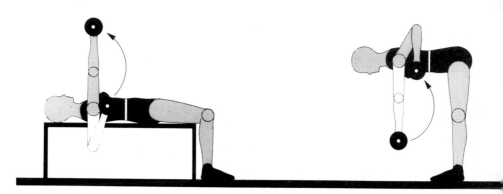

HIP FLEXION

HIP EXTENSION

TRUNK FLEXION

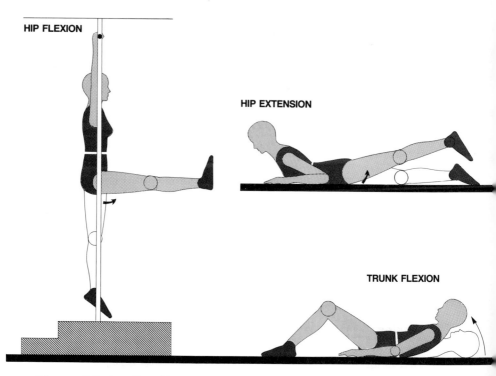

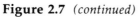

Figure 2.7 *(continued)*

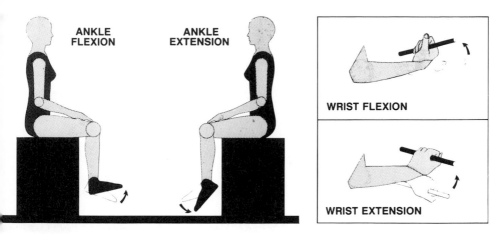

Figure 2.7 *(continued)*

Shoulder Horizontal Flexion: Decreasing the angle between the arm and the chest (forward movement with the arms at right angles to the chest).

Shoulder Horizontal Extension: Increasing the angle between the arm and the chest (backward movement with the arms at right angles to the chest).

Hip Flexion: Decreasing the angle between the thigh and the torso.

Hip Extension: Increasing the angle between the thigh and the torso.

Trunk Flexion: Decreasing the angle between the chest and the abdomen.

Ankle Flexion: Decreasing the angle between the foot and the leg.

Ankle Extension: Increasing the angle between the foot and the leg.

Wrist Flexion: Decreasing the angle between the palm and the underside of the forearm.

Wrist Extension: Increasing the angle between the palm and the underside of the forearm.

Three

Strength Training Performance Factors

There are several factors besides the physiological properties of muscle tissue that influence one's effective muscle strength. These include biomechanical factors, size factors, sex factors, age factors, training experience, training technique, and training specificity. It is important to understand how each of these factors may affect one's strength potential, and to use this information in designing and evaluating personal strength training programs.

Biomechanical Factors

It is quite possible for two persons who have developed the same amount of muscle tension to differ significantly in the amount of weight they can lift, because human movement is dependent upon a system of levers involving the long bones, joints, and muscles. The long bones act as levers, the joints serve as axes of rotation, and the skeletal muscles produce forces of sufficient magnitude to overcome resistance and control movement.

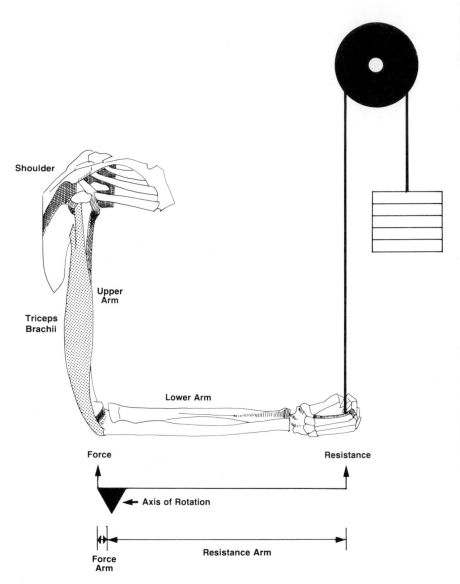

Figure 3.1 The triceps muscle operates as a first-class lever during elbow extension, because the axis of rotation is between the movement force and the resistance

First-Class Levers

In first-class levers, the axis of rotation is between the movement force and the resistive force. As shown in figure 3.1, the triceps muscle operates as a first-class lever because the elbow (axis of rotation) is between the triceps insertion (movement force) and the weightstack cable (resistive force).

Second-Class Levers

Levers of the second class place the resistive force between the axis of rotation and the movement force. Most muscles that cross two joints function as second-class levers at the first joint. For example, the quadriceps muscles cross both the hip joint (hip flexion) and the knee joint (knee extension). Because a resistive force applied to the thigh is between the first joint axis (hip) and the movement force (quadriceps insertion in leg), the quadriceps function as a second-class lever with respect to hip flexion.

Third-Class Levers

In third-class levers, the movement force is between the axis of rotation and the resistive force. As illustrated in figure 3.2, the biceps muscle serves as a third-class lever because the biceps insertion (movement force) is between the elbow (axis of rotation) and the dumbbell (resistive force).

The distance between the axis of rotation and the movement force is called the force arm, and the distance between the axis of rotation and the resistive force is called the resistance arm. The product of the resistance times the resistance arm is equal to the product of the force times the force arm when the lever is held in a static position ($R \times RA = F \times FA$). Of course, the effective force varies throughout the range of movement due to leverage factors, such as the perpendicular distance to the line of pull. Disregarding the angle of tendon insertion and the weight of the forearm, consider how the point of tendon insertion can provide leverage advantages that profoundly influence one's effective muscle strength.

Example

John has a 12-inch forearm with a biceps insertion 0.4 inches from the elbow joint. If John can produce 300 pounds of force in his biceps muscle, how heavy a dumbbell can he hold at ninety degrees elbow flexion?

$$R \times RA = F \times FA$$

$$R = \frac{F \times FA}{RA}$$

$$R = \frac{300 \text{ Pounds} \times 0.4 \text{ Inches}}{12 \text{ Inches}}$$

$$R = 10 \text{ Pounds}$$

Example

Bob also has a 12-inch forearm, but his biceps insertion is 0.6 inches from the elbow joint. If Bob can likewise produce 300 pounds of force in his biceps muscle, how heavy a dumbbell can he hold at ninety degrees elbow flexion?

$$R \times RA = F \times FA$$

$$R = \frac{F \times FA}{RA}$$

$$R = \frac{300 \text{ Pounds} \times 0.6 \text{ Inches}}{12 \text{ Inches}}$$

$$R = 15 \text{ Pounds}$$

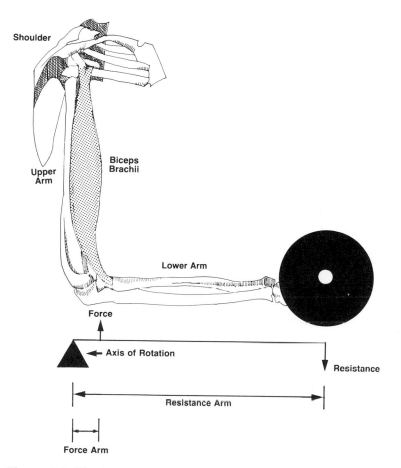

Figure 3.2 The biceps muscle operates as a third-class lever during elbow flexion. The movement force is between the axis of rotation and the resistance

In these examples Bob's maximum biceps tension of 300 pounds is equal to John's. However, due to a biceps insertion that is more favorable with respect to movement force, Bob can hold a heavier dumbbell (15 pounds versus 10 pounds) at ninety degrees elbow flexion.

These examples also demonstrate that first-class lever systems require relatively large amounts of muscle force to overcome relatively small amounts of resistive force. Although this is a disadvantage with respect to movement force, it is an advantage with respect to movement speed.

Size Factors

While biomechanical factors have an influence on one's ability to lift heavy weights, the contractile strength of a muscle is most clearly related to its cross-sectional size. Although there is considerable variation due to fiber type and fiber arrangement, most muscles produce about one to two kilograms of contractile force per square centimeter of cross-sectional area (Lamb 1978). It therefore stands to reason that the larger the cross-sectional area, the greater total force the muscle can exert.

The cross-sectional area of one's muscle is initially determined by heredity, and a large-framed individual is likely to have larger muscles than a small-framed person. However, strength training can increase the cross-sectional size of a muscle by adding contractile proteins, actin and myosin. Because there is little evidence that strength training can increase the total number of muscle fibers in humans, it is generally agreed that greater muscle size results from enlargement, not proliferation, of individual muscle fibers (Atherton et al. 1981; MacDougall 1985b). The increase in muscle size that results from strength training is called hypertrophy. Conversely, the decrease in muscle size that occurs when strength training is discontinued is known as atrophy.

The length of the muscle belly may also be an important factor with respect to muscle size (see figure 3.3). The muscle belly represents the actual muscle length between the tendon attachments. Other things being equal, it is assumed that the person with a longer muscle belly has the potential to develop greater muscle size and strength than the person with a shorter muscle belly. The length of the muscle belly appears to be an inherited characteristic that cannot be changed through training. Most people have a mixture of long-bellied muscles, medium-bellied muscles, and short-bellied muscles. Those rare individuals who possess a large percentage of long-bellied muscles are most likely to be successful in weightlifting and bodybuilding competition.

Sex Factors

Women who engage in strength training programs develop muscular strength at about the same rate as men. Research by Westcott (1974, 1976, 1979a) indicates that both males and females can increase the strength of their bench press muscles (pectoralis major,

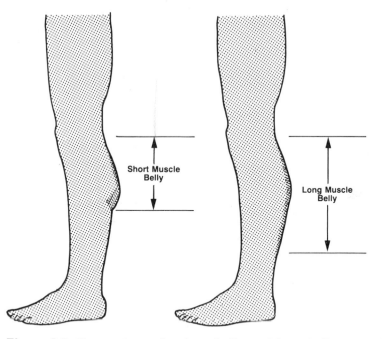

Figure 3.3 Comparison of a short-belly and long-belly gastrocnemius muscle. The length of the muscle belly may affect the potential size and strength of a muscle.

anterior deltoid, and triceps) by 3 percent to 6 percent per week, over a period of several weeks. It is also known that males and females do not differ in strength per square centimeter of muscle tissue. However, with respect to muscle size and effective muscle strength, there are definite sex-related differences. Although males and females gain strength at similar rates, postpubescent males begin with larger muscles, which provides a significant strength advantage. Furthermore, strength training increases muscle size to a greater degree in males than in females. The reason appears to be related to the male sex hormone testosterone, which plays a major role in muscle growth and hypertrophy.

By virtue of their genetic make-up, males have a greater potential for muscle size and strength than females. Nonetheless, most females can develop lower body strength that compares favorably to males on a pound-for-pound basis. Westcott (1986i) evaluated 900 adults on a Nautilus Leg Extension machine. The average male performed ten strict repetitions with 62 percent of his bodyweight, and the average female performed ten strict repetitions with 55 percent of her bodyweight.

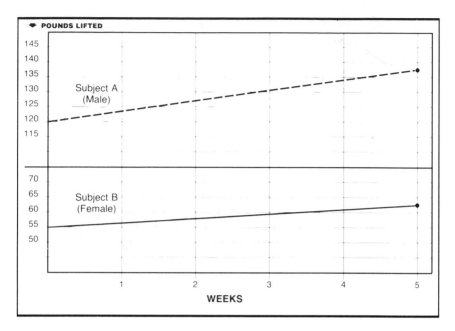

Figure 3.4 Increase in bench press strength as indicated by actual amount of weight lifted. (Bodyweights: male = 160 lbs., female = 95 lbs.)

Figures 3.4 and 3.5 illustrate the strength development of a typical college-aged male and college-aged female over a five-week training period utilizing the bench press exercise. As shown in figure 3.4 the male subject increased his bench press by twenty pounds during the training period, and the female subject increased her bench press by ten pounds. When examined in terms of percentage improvement, however, both subjects gained strength at about the same rate, approximately 4 percent per week (see figure 3.5). It appears that females may obtain the same strength benefits as males from participation in sound strength training programs.

Age Factors

Males and females gain strength through the process of maturation. However, unless they engage in strength training activities, their strength begins to decrease after age twenty. This phenomenon is not irreversible, as evidenced by the large number of older

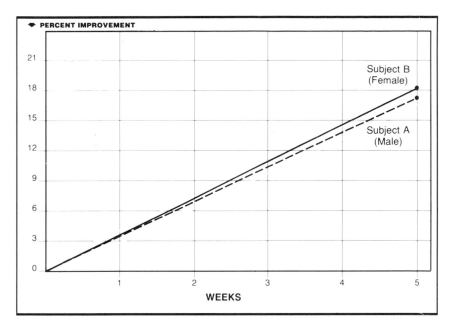

Figure 3.5 Increase in bench press strength as indicated by percent improvement. (Bodyweights: male = 160 lbs., female = 95 lbs.)

Table 3.1 Rates of strength development for female subjects of different ages (N = 14)

Age group	Average strength increase percent per week
9–13.5 years	6.4
13.5–19 years	4.7
19–27 years	2.6

weightlifting record holders and bodybuilding champions. The key to strength improvement at any age is progressive strength training. However, research (Westcott 1979a) indicates that the rate of strength development may be related to age factors (see table 3.1). Westcott compared the average weekly strength gains for three groups of female subjects (N = 14) training with the bench press exercise. One group consisted of young girls under 13.5 years of age. On the average, the girls in this group increased their strength by 6.4 percent per week. A second group was composed of older girls between 13.5

and 19 years of age. The mean strength improvement for this group was 4.7 percent per week. The third group was made up of young women over the age of 19, and the mean strength gain in this group was 2.6 percent per week.

These data suggest that strength may be developed more rapidly in younger females than in older females. Research by Sewall and Micheli (1986) and Weltman et al. (1986) indicates the preadolescent males also experience significant strength gains as a result of systematic strength training. It is therefore suggested that strength training may be more effective during periods of physical growth and maturation.

It should be noted that the older females (over age nineteen) in Westcott's 1979a study gained strength at about the same rate as the college age males in Westcott's 1974 study. Although persons of all ages can improve muscle strength, older individuals seem to increase strength more slowly than their younger counterparts.

Training Experience

Training experience implies the length of time one has been involved in a strength training program. Generally speaking, the person who has trained regularly for two years will make smaller strength gains than the person who has trained for only two weeks. During the early stages of a strength training program, improvement usually comes quickly due to motor learning factors (see chapter 4). As one's strength approaches his genetic potential, increases are much smaller and less frequent. In fact, progress appears to slow considerably during the first three months of training (Westcott 1985a, 1985c). Figure 3.6 illustrates a typical strength improvement curve over a three-month training period. Although the participant achieves a 40 percent strength gain during the first month, the strength increase is only 10 percent during the second month, and about 2.5 percent during the third month.

The process of expending more and more effort and experiencing less and less improvement can be discouraging. It is therefore important to use training experience in the most productive manner possible. First, it must be understood that if one continues to do the same exercise routine progress will plateau after several weeks.

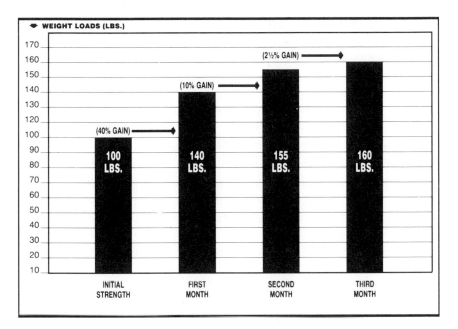

Figure 3.6 Sample three-month improvement for athlete with initial leg extension weightload of 100 lbs

Second, due to the motor learning and skill specificity aspects of muscular activity, a change in exercise is usually accompanied by a higher rate of performance improvement (see chapter 5).

Consequently, experienced strength trainers should routinely alter their training program in order to observe progress and maintain motivation. For example, Bill has been unable to complete more than ten repetitions with 150 pounds in the leg extension exercise. Rather than remain on a plateau in this exercise, he replaces leg extensions with squats. By so doing, he continues to train the quadriceps muscles, but the movement pattern is different enough to require a new neuromuscular response. The result is noticeable performance improvement in the squat exercise due to both motor learning factors and muscle development. When progress in the squat plateaus, Bill returns to the leg extension exercise. After a few training sessions he surpasses his previous performance level in this exercise, and continues to make progress.

In summary, experienced strength training participants are less likely to see regular progress because they are closer to their strength potential. By frequently changing exercises, they can continue to make performance improvements, which stimulates strength development and enhances training motivation.

Training Technique

Training technique may have a profound influence on strength development and injury prevention. For example, John can curl only 75 pounds in strict form because his biceps are not assisted by larger muscle groups. However, John can cheat curl 150 pounds by bending forward and using his large hip extensor muscles to give the barbell upward momentum.

In the first case, John uses a slow lifting movement characterized by consistent application of biceps force throughout the range of motion. This technique provides excellent stimulus for the biceps muscles and poses little risk of injury.

In the second case, John uses a fast lifting movement characterized by explosive involvement of assisting muscle groups and momentum. High levels of biceps force are required to overcome inertia at the beginning of the movement, but little biceps force is required throughout the remaining range of motion. Although this technique provides some stimulus to the biceps muscles, it places greater stress on the connective tissue and carries a higher risk of injury (Finamore 1989).

In the author's opinion, John will achieve better results by performing strict curls with 75 pounds than by performing cheat curls with 150 pounds. Generally speaking, the use of assisting muscle groups and momentum reduces the training stimulus to the target muscle group.

Another aspect of training technique is the resetting of neuromuscular inhibition levels as a result of regular practice (Ikai and Steinhaus 1961). That is, the safety mechanisms responsible for prohibiting maximum force production may be adjusted through exercise familiarity, thereby enabling the exerciser to use a greater percentage of his potential strength.

It should also be noted that a muscle produces greater tension when it is stretched just prior to contraction. For example, a standing long jump is initiated by a quick sitting movement to prestretch the thigh muscles so that they can contract more forcefully. Likewise, when one quickly lowers the bar just before the upward phase of bench press additional force can be exerted as a result of the pre-stretch.

It would appear that the stretch reflex and the elastic properties of muscle tissue are largely responsible for the greater contractile strength associated with prestretching movements. However, because quick movements with heavy weightloads may increase the risk of injury, the author does not recommend prestretching as a standard strength training technique.

Training Specificity

People frequently equate hard work with success, but this is only true when there is a strong relationship between the work being done and the desired outcomes. Both a ten-mile run and three sets of heavy squats are hard work, but the physiological responses to each type of exercise are quite different. Both the serious distance runner and the serious weightlifter may train an hour or more each day, but their physical appearances are strikingly dissimilar. Training that involves long periods of low-intensity exercise may develop cardiovascular endurance but does not improve muscle strength. Conversely, training that involves short periods of high-intensity exercise develops muscle strength but may not improve cardiovascular endurance. Experiments with laboratory animals (Gordon 1967) indicate that endurance training produces an increase in endurance enzymes, but a decrease in contractile proteins, and that strength training produces an increase in contractile proteins, but a decrease in endurance enzymes.

One should train in a specific manner to obtain specific results: strength training for muscle development and endurance training for cardiovascular development. Figure 3.7 indicates the approximate positions of various activities along the strength-endurance continuum. Note that strength-related activities are of relatively high intensity and short duration, whereas endurance-related activities are of relatively low intensity and long duration.

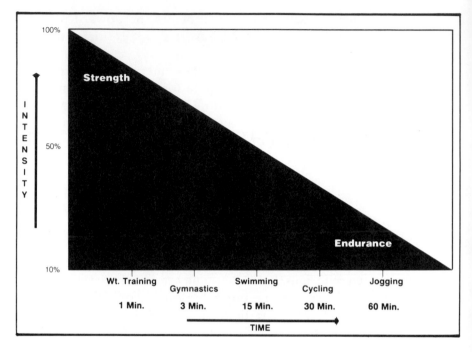

Figure 3.7 Position of various activities along the strength-endurance continuum. Note that strength-related activities are of relatively high intensity and short duration.

Four

Strength Training Research

During the past few years, the author has been privileged to conduct several research studies on strength training. This chapter will present the results of these and other investigations on the following topics: (1) research on strength training variables, including training frequency, training sets, training repetitions, training speed, training time, and activity order; and (2) research on strength training effects, including blood pressure response, heart rate response, cardiovascular response, muscle response, body composition response, and youth response.

Most of the studies presented in this chapter were conducted with average men, women, boys, and girls. The results are therefore most generalizable to average people who seek higher levels of strength fitness. The research findings may not be applicable to highly trained athletes such as competitive bodybuilders and weightlifters.

Research on Strength Training Variables

Training Frequency

Many people in our fast-paced society have difficulty maintaining a regular training schedule. While most strength training proponents advocate an every-other-day work-rest sequence, not everyone can follow this training pattern. Some enthusiasts find a few minutes every day for a short workout, while others endure a lengthy training session once or twice a week.

Table 4.1   Effects of different training frequencies on the
development of muscle strength (N = 55)

Group	(N)	Repetitions per training session	Training sessions per week	Repetitions per week	Mean percent increase
A	16	60	1	60	19%
B	20	30	2	60	17%
C	13	20	3	60	24%
D	6	12	5	60	21%

Consider one study (Westcott 1974) that compared different frequencies of training on strength development. In an attempt to isolate the frequency variable, total training workloads were equated on a weekly basis. More specifically, all fifty-five subjects performed sixty repetitions per week with the bench press exercise. Group A trained one day per week and completed all sixty repetitions (twelve sets of five reps) in a single session. Group B trained two days per week, and completed thirty repetitions (six sets of five reps) each session. Group C trained three days per week, and performed twenty repetitions (four sets of five reps) each session. Group D trained five days per week and executed twelve repetitions (two sets of six reps) each session. Table 4.1 presents the training protocols followed by the four experimental groups.

All of the subjects were tested for maximum bench press strength (1 RM) at the beginning and every 2½ weeks during the 7½ week training period. As presented in table 4.1, the subjects made excellent strength gains in the bench press exercise. However, statistical analyses showed no significant differences among the four training groups. That is, all of the training frequencies appeared equally effective for improving bench press strength. These results seem to indicate that a variety of training frequencies may be acceptable for strength development.

Summary

Based on the findings of this study it would appear that to some degree training frequency may be a matter of individual preference. Although the one day per week and five days per week training programs produced significant strength gains, the author recommends two or three evenly spaced training sessions per week as a sound strength training guideline.

Training Sets

There is little agreement as to how many sets of exercise one should perform for best strength results. Bodybuilders typically execute multiple sets with each exercise, whereas many adult fitness centers advocate a single set training policy.

DeLorme-Watkins Program

Following World War II, Thomas DeLorme and Arthur Watkins experimented with strength training for purposes of muscle rehabilitation. Their work produced one of the first systematic and progressive weight training programs to receive approval from both medical and physical education professionals. Although performed under clinical conditions, they obtained excellent results by using three sets of ten repetitions each.

The first set of ten repetitions is performed with 50 percent of the heaviest weightload that can be lifted ten times and serves as a first-level warm-up. The second set of ten repetitions is conducted with 75 percent of the heaviest weightload that can be lifted ten times and serves as a second-level warm-up. The final set of ten repetitions is executed with the heaviest weightload that can be lifted ten times and is the actual stimulus for strength development. The heaviest weightload that can be lifted ten times is called the ten repetition maximum (10 RM) weightload.

Example

The heaviest weightload that John can press ten times in succession (10-RM weightload) is 100 pounds. According to the DeLorme-Watkins training formula, John should do the following workout.

First Set:	ten repetitions with 50 pounds.
Second Set:	ten repetitions with 75 pounds.
Third Set:	ten repetitions with 100 pounds.

As John's muscles respond to the training stimulus he will be able to complete more than ten repetitions with 100 pounds. De-Lorme and Watkins recommended that a new 10-RM weightload be established when the exerciser can perform fifteen repetitions with the previous 10-RM weightload. This ensures gradual and progressive loading of the muscles in accordance with the stress adaptation principle. This program represents what is generally known as a double progressive training approach, because the exerciser alternately increases the exercise repetitions and the exercise resistance.

The Berger Program

Beginning in 1962, Richard Berger conducted several studies involving different combinations of sets and repetitions. One of Berger's first experiments (1962b) dealt with the optimum number of repetitions one should perform when training with a single set. His findings indicated that one set of the 4-RM, 6-RM, or 8-RM weightload produced greater strength gains than one set of the 2-RM, 10-RM, or 12-RM weightload. He therefore concluded that training with three to nine repetitions encompassed the optimum number of repetitions for increasing strength when training with one set, three times weekly.

Berger's best-known study (1962a) compared all combinations of one, two, and three sets with two, six, and ten repetitions per set. The results of this study suggested that three sets of six repetitions each with the 6-RM weightload was the most effective training stimulus for gaining muscular strength. Although subsequent investigations by Berger (1963) and O'Shea (1966) did not confirm the superiority of this training program, three sets of six repetitions became a very popular training format, particularly for beginners and noncompetitive weight trainers.

EXAMPLE

The heaviest weightload that Mary can curl six times in succession (6-RM weightload) is fifty pounds. According to the Berger training format, Mary should perform the following workout.

First Set:	six repetitions with 50 pounds.
Second Set:	six repetitions with 50 pounds.
Third Set:	six repetitions with 50 pounds.

When Mary begins training with the 6-RM weightload, she will probably execute fewer than six repetitions in the second and third sets due to the cumulative effects of fatigue. However, as her strength increases, she will be able to complete six repetitions in all three sets. At that time the weightload should be increased by 5 percent and the strength building process begun anew. Like the DeLorme-Watkins program, the Berger system utilizes a three-day-per-week training schedule.

The Pyramid Program

Westcott (1979a) compared the training effects of the DeLorme-Watkins system and the Berger system, along with a third program that involved three sets with increasing weightloads and decreasing repetitions. The latter is a type of pyramid program, because successive sets are done with more weight and fewer repetitions. The pyramid program was based on the exerciser's 1-RM weightload, that is, the heaviest weightload that could be lifted one time. The first set consisted of ten repetitions with 55 percent of the 1-RM weightload, the second set required five repetitions with 75 percent of the 1-RM weightload, and the third set was a single lift with 95 percent of the 1-RM weightload.

Example

The heaviest weightload that Susan can bench press once (1-RM weightload) is 100 pounds. According to Westcott's training protocol, Susan would perform the following workout.

First Set:	ten repetitions with 55 pounds.
Second Set:	five repetitions with 75 pounds.
Third Set:	one repetition with 95 pounds.

The pyramid program is similar to the DeLorme-Watkins program in that both involve two progressively heavier warm-up sets and one set designed to produce the training effect. They are different with respect to the relative amount of resistance used for the training stimulus in the final set.

Table 4.2 Improvement in bench press performance by groups training with Berger, DeLorme-Watkins, and pyramid programs (N = 14)

Group	Berger	DeLorme-Watkins	Pyramid
Subjects	5	4	5
Mean Improvement/week	3.7%	4.3%	4.3%

Program Comparison

All of the participants in Westcott's study improved their bench press performance, and the rates of strength development for the three training groups were quite similar. Comparative results of the DeLorme-Watkins system, the Berger system, and the pyramid program are summarized in table 4.2. Because there were no statistically significant differences in strength gains among the three training groups, it would appear that these training programs may be equally effective for developing muscle strength.

Single Sets versus Multiple Sets

The author conducted two studies examining the effects of single sets and multiple sets on strength development. The first study (Westcott 1986j) compared training with one, two, and three sets of exercise on Nautilus equipment. Due to injuries, illnesses, and dropouts, the number of subjects who completed the three-set program was too small to include in the data analyses. Consequently, this study actually compared twenty-two subjects who performed one high-intensity set of exercise with twenty-two other subjects who performed two high-intensity sets of exercise. The exercises used in this study were the Leg Extension, Leg Curl, Torso Pullover, Arm Extension, and Arm Curl.

As illustrated in table 4.3, the results showed no statistically significant differences in strength development between the subjects who performed one set of each exercise and the subjects who performed two sets of each exercise.

The second study (Westcott et al. 1989) differed from the first by using a larger number of subjects (seventy-seven men and women), a longer training duration (ten weeks), and bodyweight exercises (dips and chins).

Table 4.3 Improvement in Nautilus performance by groups training with one and two sets per exercise (N = 44)

Group	One set	Two set
Subjects	22	22
Mean improvement per/week (5 exercises)	15.8%	15.0%

To enable the subjects to complete the prescribed number of dips and chins in their exercise protocol, all training was performed on a computerized air-pressure apparatus that lifted a given percentage of the exerciser's bodyweight during each dip and chin. The Gravitron machine was individually programmed so that each participant experienced muscle failure at the end of his/her training session.

Each subject selected one of the following exercise protocols and trained in this manner throughout the study. Whenever the subject could complete his/her specific training program with a given resistance, the level of machine assistance was reduced slightly to make the workout more demanding.

EXAMPLE

1 set × 5 reps	2 sets × 5 reps	3 sets × 5 reps
1 set × 10 reps	2 sets × 10 reps	3 sets × 10 reps
1 set × 15 reps	2 sets × 15 reps	3 sets × 15 reps

Example: A subject in the two sets of ten reps group would perform ten dips and ten chins, followed by ten more dips and ten more chins.

Before their first training session and after their last (thirtieth) training session, all subjects were tested for the maximum number of dips and chins they could perform in strict technique with their full bodyweight. The total number of dips and chins correctly completed determined the subject's pretraining and posttraining scores.

As illustrated in table 4.4, all of the training groups made excellent improvements in their dips and chins performance. There were no statistically significant differences among the subjects who performed one set of each exercise, the subjects who did two sets of

Table 4.4 Improvement in dips and chins performance by groups training with one, two, and three sets per exercise (N = 77)

Group	One set	Two sets	Three sets
Subjects	10	35	32
Mean improvement	4.8 Reps	4.1 Reps	5.2 Reps

each exercise, and the subjects who did three sets of each exercise. As a side note, there were also no statistically significant differences among the groups training with five, ten, or fifteen repetitions per set.

Summary

Based on the results of these studies on training sets, it would appear that the number of exercise sets one performs has little affect on strength development. It seems that the essential stimulus for gaining strength is one high-intensity set of resistive exercise. Performing additional sets of exercise appears neither advantageous nor disadvantageous as measured by improvement in strength performance.

In terms of training effectiveness, the author does not favor one-set, two-set, or three-set training as all seem to be equally useful for strength development. However, in terms of training efficiency, single set training appears to accomplish the same strength results in much less time.

Training Repetitions

There is an inverse relationship between the weightload utilized for a particular exercise and the number of repetitions that can be executed. When one uses the heaviest weightload possible, only a single lift can be performed. As the weightload is reduced, more repetitions can be completed. However, Berger (1965) found that training with less than 65 percent of maximum weightload may not be effective for strength development.

Between 1948 and 1970, a considerable amount of research was conducted to determine the optimum number of repetitions for developing muscle strength with isotonic training. DeLorme and Watkins (1948) advocated an exercise program based on ten repetitions per set.

Berger (1962a) compared nine different strength training programs involving all combinations of one, two, and three sets with two, six, and ten repetitions, and found that three sets of six repetitions produced the greatest strength gains. Berger (1962b) reported the results of another study in which one set of three to nine repetitions proved equally effective for strength improvement.

In a 1963 investigation, Berger found no significant differences among training programs utilizing two, six, or ten repetitions per set. O'Shea (1966) also found no significant differences among training programs using two and three repetitions, five and six repetitions, or nine and ten repetitions. In a similar study, Withers (1970) found no significant differences among training programs incorporating three, five, or seven repetitions per set.

During the seventies, Nautilus literature had a major impact on strength training protocols, and eight to twelve repetitions became standard procedure for many strength training participants (Darden 1977).

Westcott conducted two studies comparing eight-repetition training and twelve-repetition training. The subjects who trained with eight repetitions used the heaviest weightload that could be performed eight times, and the subjects who trained with twelve repetitions used the heaviest weightload that could be performed twelve times. The first study (1986j) showed no differences between the two training groups, but the second study (1986h) revealed better results with eight-repetition training.

Jones (1986) conducted a considerable amount of research in the area of muscle endurance. He found that subjects with low muscle endurance required only four or five isokinetic repetitions to reduce their starting strength by 25 percent, while subjects with high muscle endurance required fifteen to sixteen isokinetic repetitions to reduce their starting strength by 25 percent. Jones suggested that the differences in muscle endurance may be due to inherent physiological characteristics that are not altered by training. If Jones' hypothesis were correct, it might partly account for the inconsistent findings with regards to optimum training repetitions.

Westcott (1986l) examined differences in muscle performance with a given submaximum resistance. The eighty-seven subjects (forty-nine men and thirty-eight women) were tested on a Nautilus 10-Degree Chest machine to determine the heaviest weightload that they could perform one time. After a five-minute rest, the participants completed as many strict repetitions as possible with 75 percent of their maximum weightload.

The findings of this study showed that most subjects performed 8–13 repetitions with 75 percent of their maximum weightload (see figure 4.1). As shown in table 4.5, the mean score for all subjects was 10.8 repetitions. However, it was also apparent that the subjects varied considerably in the number of repetitions they could complete with a given percentage of their maximum resistance. Two subjects completed only 5 repetitions, while one subject performed 24 repetitions with the same relative resistance.

It would therefore appear that some people have high levels of muscle endurance while others have low levels of muscle endurance. Because all of the subjects exercised regularly with one set of eight to twelve repetitions, their relative muscle endurance would seem to be independent of the training procedures.

These findings tend to support Jones' (1986) contention that performance differences with the same relative resistance are due to inherent physiological characteristics. It is possible that differences in muscle fiber types may be a major factor in the number of repetitions one can complete with a given submaximum weightload.

Summary

As a result of widely published strength training guidelines, many participants follow an eight to twelve repetition protocol. Westcott's (1986l) research indicates that this is a safe and effective training recommendation, as most people can perform eight to twelve strict repetitions with 75 percent of their maximum resistance. However, with respect to training specificity, it may be advisable for individuals with low-endurance muscles to train with fewer repetitions and for persons with high-endurance muscles to train with more repetitions.

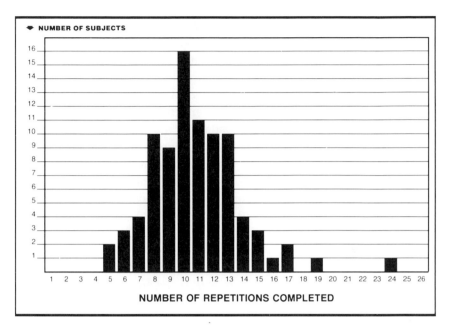

Figure 4.1 Distribution of repetitions completed with 75 percent of maximum weightload

Table 4.5 Descriptive statistics for repetitions completed with 75 percent of maximum weightload (N = 87)

		Repetitions		
Subjects	*(N)*	*Range*	*Mean*	*Standard deviation*
Male	49	5–19	10.2	2.8
Female	38	6–24	11.6	3.2
All	87	5–24	10.8	3.1

Training Speed

Perhaps the area of greatest controversy in strength training is movement speed. Advocates of fast strength training believe that fast movement speeds enhance explosive muscle power (Counsilman 1976). Conversely, proponents of slow strength training contend that slow movement speeds increase strength development and reduce injury potential (Pipes 1979).

In 1970, Moffroid and Whipple compared the effects of two movement speeds on muscle strength. One group of subjects performed an isokinetic knee extension at a speed of 36 degrees per second. Another group of subjects performed an isokinetic knee extension at a speed of 108 degrees per second. The results showed that the slower trained subjects made greater strength gains when tested at the slower speed, and that the faster trained subjects made greater strength gains when tested at the faster speed.

A study by Coyle et al. (1981) produced similar results. The slower trained subjects (60 degrees per second) showed more strength improvement at the slower speed, while the faster trained subjects (300 degrees per second) showed more strength improvement at the faster speed.

Both of these studies revealed a specificity of training effect. That is, slower training appeared to be more effective for strength development at slower speeds, and faster training appeared to be more effective for strength development at faster speeds.

Palmieri (1987) trained fifty-four subjects with squats, leg extensions, and heel raises. One group trained with slow movement speeds, another group trained with fast movement speeds, and a third group combined both slow and fast movement speeds. All of the training groups improved in leg power, but there were no significant differences with respect to the training speed. Palmieri's findings indicated that slow strength training, fast strength training, and mixed strength training (slow and fast) may be equally effective for developing power.

In an attempt to reduce hard to control variables between training groups, Westcott (1986a) conducted a study in which all subjects received both experimental treatments. Each participant trained one leg at a relatively slow speed (60 degrees per second) and the other leg at a relatively fast speed (240 degrees per second).

Six women between eighteen and thirty-six years of age served as subjects in this investigation. All of the women were healthy, physically active individuals who did not engage in any strength training activities before or during the study. Each subject was introduced to the knee extension movement on the computerized Cybex II isokinetic strength testing and training unit. After several practice trials, each leg was tested for maximum strength at 60 and 240 degrees per second.

Table 4.6 Comparison of strength gains for slow-trained leg and fast-trained leg at sixty degrees per second (N = 6)

Group	Mean initial strength	Mean final strength	Mean strength increase	Mean percent increase
Slow-trained leg	108 lbs.	118 lbs.	10 lb.	9%
Fast-trained leg	106 lbs.	105 lbs.	None	None

Table 4.7 Comparison of strength gains for slow-trained leg and fast-trained leg at 240 degrees per second (N = 6)

Group	Mean initial strength	Mean final strength	Mean strength increase	Mean percent increase
Slow-trained leg	60 lbs.	65 lbs.	5 lbs.	8%
Fast-trained leg	63 lbs.	63 lbs.	None	None

All subjects followed the same strength training protocol. Upon securing the left leg to the training apparatus, they performed twenty seconds of knee extensions at 60 degrees per second. The subjects completed three sets of exercise with a forty-second recovery period between sets. Upon securing the right leg to the training apparatus, they performed twenty seconds of knee extensions at 240 degrees per second. The subjects again completed three sets of exercise with a forty-second recovery period between sets.

After training three times per week for three weeks, each leg was retested for maximum strength at 60 and 240 degrees per second. As presented in tables 4.6 and 4.7, the slow-trained leg showed significant strength gains at both movement speeds. The fast-trained leg did not improve strength at either movement speed.

The results of this study indicated that training at 60 degrees per second may be more effective than training at 240 degrees per second for improving muscle strength at both speeds of movement.

As shown in tables 4.6 and 4.7, the subjects invariably produced higher strength outputs at the slower movement speed than at the faster movement speed. Research by Lesmes et al. (1983) determined that both fast-twitch and slow-twitch muscle fibers are activated during maximum muscle contractions regardless of the movement speed.

It is therefore suggested that more muscle force may be produced at slow movement speeds because there is more time to activate both slow-twitch and fast-twitch muscle fibers. It has also been postulated that faster movement speeds create more internal muscle friction, with a resulting decrease in force output (Jones et al. 1988).

Gettman and Ayres (1978) examined the effects of training speed on body composition. Their findings showed that subjects who trained with slow movement speeds improved body composition more than subjects who trained with fast movement speeds.

Summary

The research on training speed has not produced consistent findings. Some studies seemed to favor slower movement speeds while others found a specificity of training effect. However, all of the studies revealed slow strength training to be more effective than fast strength training when evaluated at slow movement speeds. Because slow movement speeds are characterized by greater force output, the author recommends slow strength training technique whenever possible.

Training Time

Most people feel that training time is a matter of personal preference with little bearing on one's strength development. Some people seem to function best in the morning, while others tend to be more productive in the evening. Because most sports practice sessions are held after school, athletes grow accustomed to training in the afternoon. Without exploring the area of biorhythms, it would seem to make sense that once a training schedule has been established, one will probably perform best at his or her regular workout time. However, it is also logical to assume that the cumulative effect of general fatigue may influence physical performance later in the day.

Westcott (1986j) decided to test this hypothesis on an important muscle group that typically works sixteen hours a day, even while driving the car, sitting in the office, or studying in the library. The trapezius and posterior neck muscles maintain the head in an erect

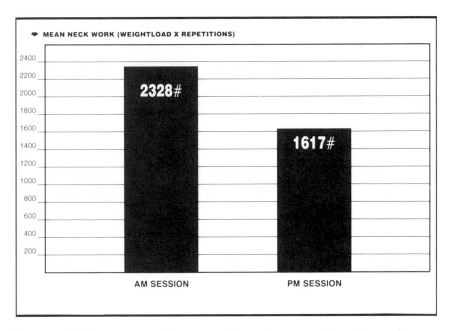

Figure 4.2 Comparison of A.M. results and P.M. results with neck extensor exercise

posture throughout one's working hours. Needless to say, the neck extensors are key muscles with regards to safety and performance in sports such as football and wrestling.

The subjects in this study were ten men and women who were already engaged in a strength training program. All of the participants had sedentary occupations that required a minimum amount of physical exertion. Each subject was evaluted for neck extension strength on a Nautilus 4-Way Neck machine with a weightload that could be lifted at least ten repetitions. The subjects were randomly tested with the same weightload before 10:00 A.M. and after 5:00 P.M. on nonconsecutive days.

The results showed that the subjects completed 44 percent more repetitions in the morning session than in the evening session (see figure 4.2). The morning performance exceeded the evening performance in every case, even though many of the subjects normally trained later in the day.

These statistically significant findings suggested that daily fatigue may have a profound effect on the neck extensor muscles. It would appear that holding one's head in an upright position for several hours a day may reduce neck strength substantially.

Summary

In accordance with the principle of rebuilding time (see chapter 5), one should take a workout at the peak of the muscle building process to obtain maximum strength benefits. Similarly, one should train when both the energy level and strength level are highest for best results. These findings indicate that the neck extensor muscles perform significantly better at the beginning of the day than at the end of the day. It is therefore recommended that neck strengthening exercises be performed during the morning hours when the general fatigue level is lower. It is possible that morning strength workouts may produce excellent overall results for the same reason, but individual training preferences should certainly be taken into consideration.

Activity Order

Consider the person who wants to combine strength training and endurance training. It is recommended that one take a hard strength workout and a hard endurance workout on the same day, followed by a recovery day.

Westcott (1986g) researched the effects of activity order on exercise performance. The subjects in this study attempted to perform two identical workouts. In one session, they first did a specific strength program (eleven Nautilus exercises), rested five minutes, and then did a specific endurance program (twenty minutes stationary cycling). In another session they first did the endurance program, rested five minutes, and then did the strength program.

As illustrated in figures 4.3 and 4.4, the activity order had a greater influence on endurance performance than on strength performance. The strength performance was essentially the same in both training protocols. However, the endurance performance produced a higher heart rate response when it followed the strength workout. That is, prior endurance exercise reduced strength performance by only 1 percent, but prior strength exercise reduced endurance performance by 8 percent.

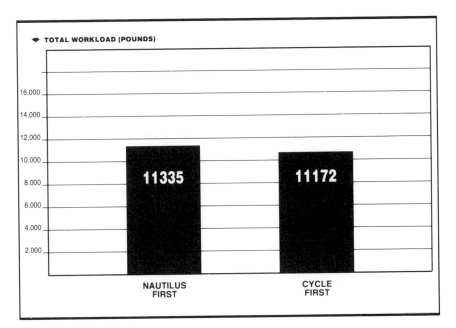

Figure 4.3 Effect of activity order on strength performance during Nautilus workout

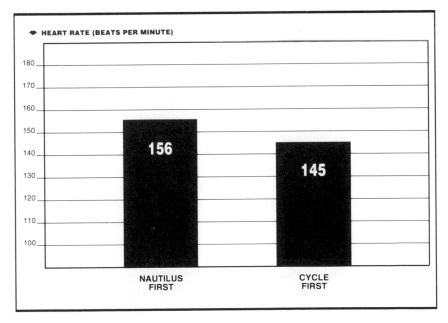

Figure 4.4 Effect of activity order on endurance performance during cycle ergometer workout

Summary

Based on these findings, it may be advisable to perform endurance training prior to strength training when both workouts are taken close together. However, because the performance differences were not great, it is recommended that personal objectives be considered when designing a training protocol.

Research on Strength Training Effects

Blood Pressure Response

There is a common misconception that strength training has an adverse affect on blood pressure. Although exercise physiologists are well aware that isometric strength training can cause unusually large increases in systolic and diastolic blood pressures, there is considerably less information on blood pressure response to non-isometric strength training (Karpovich and Sinning 1971; Mathews and Fox 1976; Astrand and Rodahl 1977; Lamb 1978; Pollock, Wilmore, and Fox 1978).

Recent studies of blood pressure changes during non-isometric strength training have produced different results. MacDougall et al. (1983) found extremely high systolic and diastolic blood pressures in bodybuilders during heavy leg exercises. In one subject the intra-arterial blood pressure measured 400/300 mm Hg. It is possible that other factors, such as essential hypertension, use of anabolic steroids, and excessive body mass, may have been at least partly responsible for the unusually high blood pressure response (Wright 1978; Hunter and McCarthy 1982).

Freedson, Chang, and Katch (1984) reported blood pressures around 240/155 mm Hg during free weight and hydraulic bench press exercises. These readings were lower than MacDougall's (1983) readings, but higher than those obtained by Westcott and Howes (1983) and Westcott (1986b).

Westcott and Howes (1983) studied blood pressure response during one-arm biceps curls with light, medium, and heavy weight-loads. Blood pressures were monitored throughout each ten-repetition exercise set by means of a sphygmomanometer and stethoscope on the nonexercising arm. The subjects were twenty-four men and women who had no medical history of cardiovascular disease.

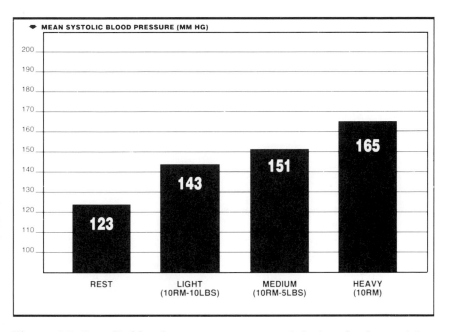

Figure 4.5 Systolic blood pressures at rest and during final repetition with light, medium, and heavy weightloads

The mean systolic blood pressure increased gradually from 123 mm Hg at rest to 165 mm Hg during the final repetition with the 10-RM weightload. The mean diastolic pressure measured 75 mm Hg both before and immediately after the exercise set. Figure 4.5 shows that the systolic blood pressure response was directly related to the training intensity. The peak systolic readings were 143 mm Hg with the light weightload, 151 mm Hg with the medium weightload, and 165 mm Hg with the heavy weightload.

Sex comparisons revealed higher peak systolic pressures for the male subjects, and age comparisons revealed higher peak systolic pressures for the subjects over thirty-eight years of age (see table 4.8).

Based on the findings of this study, it would appear that one-arm biceps curls performed with the 10-RM weightload do not produce abrupt, excessive, or unusual blood pressure responses. In fact, the 34 percent increase in systolic pressure (see figure 4.6) was similar to a 35 percent increase in systolic pressure measured on twenty-three subjects during stationary cycling (see figure 4.7).

Table 4.8 Mean systolic blood pressure responses during ten-repetition sets of one-arm dumbbell curls (N = 24)

Subjects	Resting systolic pressure	Peak systolic pressure	Percent increase
All	123	165	34%
Males	131	179	37%
Females	114	148	29%
Over 38	132	175	33%
Under 38	115	154	34%

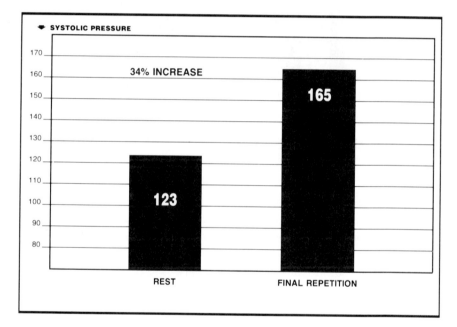

Figure 4.6 Systolic blood pressure response during 10-RM exercise set one-arm curls (N = 24)

Because lower body exercises involve more muscle mass and more muscle force than upper body exercises, Westcott (1986b) examined blood pressure response during Nautilus duo-squats with heavy weightloads. Blood pressures were monitored throughout each ten-repetition exercise set by means of a sphygmomanometer and stethoscope on the right arm. The subjects were twenty-five men and women with no medical history of cardiovascular disease.

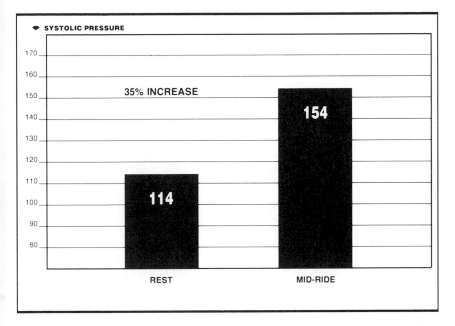

Figure 4.7 Systolic blood pressure response during stationary cycling (N = 23)

The mean systolic blood pressure increased gradually from 127 mm Hg at rest to 190 mm Hg during the final repetition with the 10-RM weightload (see figure 4.8). The mean diastolic pressure measured 73 mm Hg before and 61 mm Hg immediately after the exercise set.

Sex comparisons revealed higher peak systolic pressures for the male participants, and age comparisons revealed higher peak systolic pressures for the subjects over thirty-eight years of age (see table 4.9).

Although the Nautilus duo-squats produced a 50 percent increase in systolic blood pressure, the response pattern was similar to one-arm biceps curls. All of the subjects demonstrated a gradual, progressive, and predictable systolic pressure increase during the ten-repetition exercise sets. It is noted that a systolic pressure of 190 mm Hg is not uncommon during vigorous physical activity, and few exercises are as demanding as the Nautilus duo-squat.

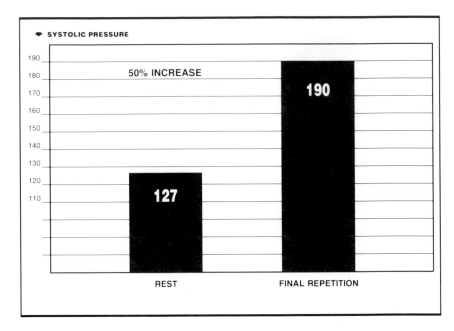

Figure 4.8 Systolic blood pressure during 10-RM exercise set Nautilus duo-squats (N = 25)

Table 4.9 Mean systolic blood pressure responses during ten-repetition sets of Nautilus duo-squats (N = 25)

Subjects	Resting systolic pressure	Peak systolic pressure	Percent increase
All	127	190	50%
Males	130	195	50%
Females	115	170	48%
Over 38	125	193	54%
Under 38	129	188	46%

Circuit Strength Training

Westcott and Pappas (1987) examined the immediate effects of circuit strength training on blood pressure. One hundred men and women participated in this study. The subjects performed one set of eight–twelve repetitions on the following Nautilus machines: (1) leg extension, (2) leg curl, (3) hip adduction, (4) hip abduction, (5) low back, (6) abdominal, (7) 10-degree chest, (8) back pullover, (9) lateral

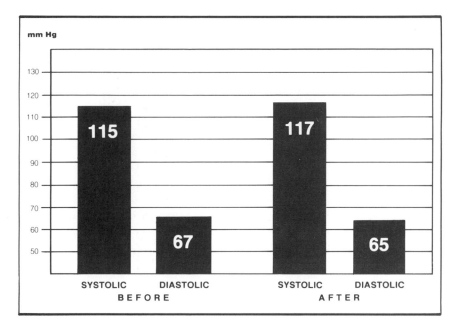

Figure 4.9 Blood pressure readings thirty–sixty seconds before and after performing an eleven-station circuit strength training session (N — 100)

raise, (10) biceps, and (11) triceps. The subjects' standing blood pressures were recorded thirty to sixty seconds before and thirty to sixty seconds after performing the eleven-station exercise circuit.

The average age of the participants was thirty-seven years and the average time for completing the strength training circuit was twenty-nine minutes. As presented in figure 4.9, the mean pre-exercise blood pressure reading was 115/67 mm Hg and the mean post-exercise blood pressure reading was 117/65 mm Hg.

These results indicated that blood pressure readings were essentially the same before and after twenty-nine minutes of circuit strength training with relatively heavy resistance. Note that the participants in this study, most of whom had performed regular circuit strength training for over a year, recorded relatively low blood pressures both before (115/67 mm Hg) and after (117/65 mm Hg) the exercise session.

Harris and Holly (1987) conducted a low resistance–high repetition circuit strength training program for borderline hypertensive individuals. Their subjects experienced a significant decrease in resting diastolic blood pressure (96 to 91 mm Hg) after nine weeks of training.

Another circuit strength training study (Hurley et al. 1988) involved healthy, middle-aged men. The findings showed a significant reduction in diastolic blood pressure (84 to 79 mm Hg) as a result of the sixteen-week resistive exercise program.

Other researchers (Stone et al. 1983; Hagberg et al. 1984) also reported reductions in resting blood pressure as a result of regular strength training.

Summary

Based on the majority of blood pressure studies reviewed, it would appear that sensible strength training does not have an adverse affect on blood pressure in healthy adults. In fact, some of the research findings suggest that regular strength training may actually elicit positive blood pressure adaptations.

Sensible strength training is characterized by continuous movement and continuous breathing throughout the exercise set. It is emphasized that prolonged isometric contractions or breath-holding can produce excessive blood pressure responses, and should therefore be avoided. It is recommended that persons with elevated resting blood pressures or other cardiovascular abnormalities consult their physician before beginning a strength training program.

Heart Rate Response

Whenever the demand for energy increases, the heart rate increases. The heart is similar to the fuel pump in an automobile, and the muscles are analogous to the engine. As the muscles perform work, the heart must pump blood to the work site to replenish energy supplies and remove metabolic waste products. Because the heart pumps blood throughout the entire body, activity in any of the major muscle groups produces a faster heart rate. Although more oxygen is consumed by larger muscle groups, the heart rate response is essentially the same for a leg extension and an arm extension (Hempel and Wells, 1985).

Westcott (1985b) found a gradual and progressive increase in heart rate during ten repetitions with the 10-RM weightload. His findings also indicated an inverse relationship between the rest in-

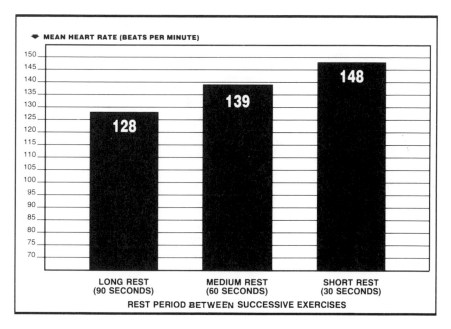

Figure 4.10 Mean peak heart rates for ten-station workout with long, medium, and short rests between successive exercises (N = 30)

terval and the heart rate response. As illustrated in figure 4.10, when the thirty subjects took ninety second rests between exercises their mean peak heart rate was 128 beats per minute. As the rest intervals decreased to sixty seconds and thirty seconds, the mean peak heart rates increased to 139 beats per minute and 148 beats per minute, respectively.

Summary

The heart rate response and systolic blood pressure response to isotonic strength training are similar in that both increase gradually, progressively, and predictably during an exercise set. The less rest taken between successive exercises, the higher the mean heart rate response. The following case study illustrates a typical heart rate and systolic blood pressure response to a ten-exercise strength training circuit.

Case Study: Heart Rate and Systolic Blood Pressure Responses to Strength Training

Subject: Mary Ellen   Age: 24   Workout Time: 19 Min.   Date: 3-31-86

		Heart Rate (BPM)	*Systolic Blood Pressure (mm Hg)*	*Double Product (HR × SBP)*
Resting Values		78	120/78	9,360
Exercise	*Repetitions*			
Leg extension	11	126	178	22,428
Leg curl	12	138	212	29,256
Hip adduction	12	112	200	22,400
Hip abduction	12	143	222	31,746
Low back	12	136	218	29,648
Abdominal	12	145	182	26,390
Pullover	10	114	178	20,292
Lateral raise	10	112	192	21,504
Biceps curl	10	110	182	20,020
Triceps extension	12	105	202	21,210
Mean exercise values		124	197	24,489
Thirty-second postexercise values		99	124/70	12,276

Cardiovascular Response

As presented in a previous section, regular strength training may cause a reduction in resting blood pressure readings (Stone et al 1983; Hagberg et al. 1984; Harris and Holly 1987; Hurley et al. 1988). There is also evidence that strength training may improve lipoprotein and lipid profiles. Several studies have shown decreases in LDL (bad) cholesterol levels (Stone et al. 1982; Johnson et al. 1982; Goldberg et al. 1984; Hurley et al. 1988), and increases in HDL (good) cholesterol levels (Johnson et al. 1982; Goldberg et al. 1984; Hurley et al. 1988).

Other investigators have reported increased left ventricle wall thickness as a result of progressive strength training (Morganroth et al. 1975; Mathews and Fox 1976; Fox 1979; Ricci et al. 1982). There are also indications that progressive strength training may increase muscle capillarization (Schantz 1982; McDonagh and Davies 1984). In addition, Peterson (1976), Stone et al. (1983), and Goldberg et al. (1983) found significant reductions in subjects' double products (heart rate × systolic blood pressure) after regular participation in a weight training program.

These findings suggest that strength training may have some positive effects on the cardiovascular system. Other studies have attempted to determine whether strength training can increase aerobic capacity (maximum oxygen consumption). Improvements in aerobic capacity are typically observed when one regularly performs over twelve minutes of endurance exercise at an intensity sufficient to keep the heart rate above 75 percent of maximum (Zohman 1974; Ward 1988).

According to Hurley et al. (1984) and Hempel and Wells (1985), even though circuit strength training can maintain relatively high heart rates, it does not use a high enough percentage of maximum oxygen uptake to produce cardiovascular adaptations. However, Messier and Dill (1985) found a significant increase in maximum oxygen consumption after ten weeks of circuit strength training. In fact, the strength program participants improved their maximum oxygen consumption as much as the subjects who participated in a running program. In a similar study, Harris and Holly (1987) found significant aerobic improvements in their subjects as a result of circuit strength training. One circuit strength training program (Keleman et al. 1986) showed significant cardiovascular improvement in cardiac rehabilitation participants, and another (Weltman et al. 1986) revealed significant aerobic increases in young boys.

Westcott and Warren (1985) conducted a high-intensity circuit strength training program in which the subjects completed one set of eight to fifteen repetitions on ten Nautilus machines with only fifteen seconds rest between exercises. After four weeks of training, the subjects' mean performance on a standard cycle ergometer test improved by 19 percent (see figure 4.11). Because the ability to perform cycle ergometer exercise is related to both cardiovascular endurance and muscular strength, the subjects' 52 percent increase in muscle strength may have been largely responsible for their better score on the posttraining assessment.

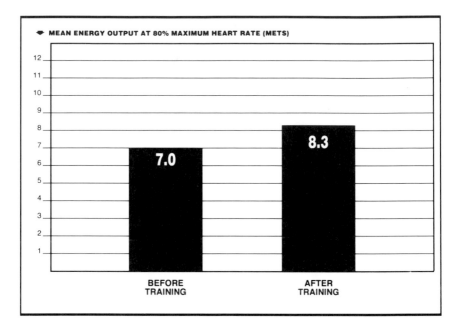

Figure 4.11 Energy output in Mets at 80 percent of maximum heart rate before and after circuit strength training program (N = 6)

Summary

It is well-established that rhythmic, endurance exercise such as jogging, cycling, and swimming are the preferred means for cardio-vascular conditioning. However, there is evidence that strength training (especially circuit strength training) may provide several positive cardiovascular effects. These include reduced resting blood pressure, improved lipoprotein and lipid profile, increased left ventricle wall thickness, increased muscle capillarization, reduced double products, and enhanced aerobic capacity.

Muscle Response

Most people who begin a strength fitness program are encouraged by the relatively large strength gains they experience during the first few weeks of training. Beginners may increase their strength by more than 40 percent after one month of regular workouts (Westcott 1984a; Westcott and Warren 1985). Unfortunately, the rate of improvement tends to drop off sharply during the second month of training.

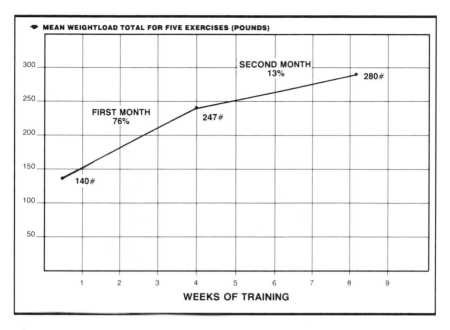

Figure 4.12 Percentage improvement during first and second months of strength training (N = 6)

Westcott (1985c) observed six female subjects during eight weeks of supervised strength training. The subjects were evaluated for muscle strength (10 RM) at the beginning, midpoint, and end of the training program. All participants performed five exercises, three days per week throughout the course of the study.

As illustrated in figure 4.12, the women increased their overall muscle strength 76 percent during the first month, and 13 percent during the second month. Although the subjects made 100 percent improvement after eight weeks of training, most of the strength gain occurred during the first month.

Palmieri (1987) obtained similar results with a ten-week training program for the leg muscles. The subjects improved their squat performance by 16 percent during the first six weeks, but only 5 percent over the following four weeks.

Fukunaga (1976) found a 60 percent strength increase during the first three weeks of training, but only a 30 percent strength increase over the next six weeks. His results also revealed no increase in muscle cross-sectional area after the first three weeks of training, but a 9 percent increase in muscle cross-sectional area during the next six weeks.

Westcott (1985c) compared performance improvement on selected weight training machines to strength gains measured on computerized strength testing equipment. The subjects were tested for maximum leg extension strength and maximum leg flexion strength on a Cybex II isokinetic apparatus. They were also tested for the ten-repetition maximum weightload (10-RM) on a Nautilus Leg Extension machine and Nautilus Leg Curl machine. The subjects trained three days per week for four weeks. The training protocol was one set of eight to twelve repetitions on each of the Nautilus machines, with a 5 percent weight increase whenever twelve repetitions were completed. Two days after the final training session, the subjects were again evaluated for maximum leg extension strength and maximum leg flexion strength on the Cybex II apparatus. The same movement pattern and movement speed (sixty degrees per second) were used in all of the testing and training sessions.

As shown in figure 4.13, the performance improvements observed on the Nautilus machines were much greater than the strength gains determined by the computerized strength tests. The subjects increased their ten-repetition maximum weightloads by about 70 percent but improved their maximum isokinetic strength by less than 10 percent.

The findings of these studies indicate that factors other than muscle development may have been partly responsible for the subjects' large performance improvements. It has been suggested that much of the early performance improvement may be due to motor learning factors (McDonagh and Davies 1984). Fleck and Kraemer (1987) describe this phenomenon as a more efficient recruitment pattern of the muscle fibers.

It would appear that initial performance improvement is influenced more by better utilization of available muscle tissue than by development of new muscle tissue (Ikai and Fukunaga 1970; Moritani and DeVries 1979; Hakkinen and Komi 1983). Conversely, motor learning factors probably play a less significant role in subsequent performance improvement, and the smaller gains attained later in the training program more likely represent new muscle development.

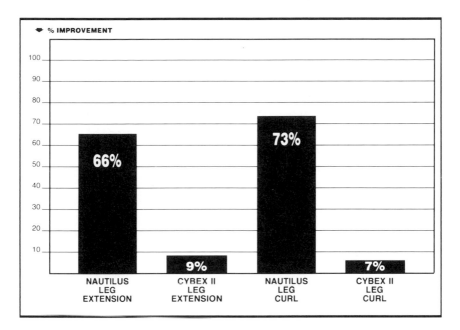

Figure 4.13 Comparison of strength improvement on Nautilus exercises and Cybex II tests (N = 3)

Summary

Most strength training participants experience relatively large increases in their performance levels during the first months of training. Research indicates that much of the initial performance improvement is due to motor learning factors, as practice enhances neurological efficiency and enables the exerciser to use available muscle tissue more effectively. Subsequent strength gains come more slowly but are largely due to the development of new muscle tissue.

Body Composition Response

Body composition refers to the ratio of fat weight to lean weight (bones, organs, muscle, etc.). Many fitness authorities (Myers 1975; Golding et al. 1982) recommend that males should be about 15 percent fat and females should be about 20 percent fat. Improvements in body composition can be attained by gaining lean weight (muscle), losing fat weight, or both.

Katch and Drumm (1986) summarized several studies in which strength training produced positive changes in body composition (Misner et al. 1974; Wilmore 1974; Pipes and Wilmore 1975; Pipes 1978). Each of these studies involved eight to ten weeks of regular strength exercise and increased lean weight by 1 to 3 pounds (2.3 pounds mean increase).

Although adding muscle weight is an excellent means for improving body composition, losing fat weight is a more popular approach. If asked how to best reduce fat weight, most people would suggest a low-calorie diet. Unfortunately, research indicates that cutting calories without exercise has some undesirable effects. One result of dieting alone is a decrease in metabolic rate (Clark 1985). Apparently, the body adapts to fewer food calories by slowing down its rate of energy production. Another result of dieting alone is a loss of lean weight including muscle tissue, organ tissue, and extracellular fluid (Darden 1981). It seems that when the caloric supply is diminished, the body draws upon both fat sources and functional tissue for energy requirements.

Most physiologists, nutritionists, and physicians agree that a sensible exercise program should accompany a sound reducing diet for best results. Exercise tends to maintain one's normal metabolic rate and lessen the loss of lean tissue. In addition, exercise utilizes calories, which facilitates fat reduction. However, the type of exercise one performs may have considerable bearing on physiological responses.

Many people believe that aerobic activity is best for losing fat because it burns large amounts of calories. Jogging, bicycling, and swimming may consume an additional 10–15 calories per minute while one is exercising (Astrand and Rodahl 1977). However, shortly after the exercise session, one's metabolism returns to normal (Clark 1985). A twenty-minute run would therefore use about 200–300 more calories per day than performing no exercise.

Strength training may be a more effective means for losing fat because it increases calorie utilization while one is exercising and also while one is at rest. That is, the additional muscle developed through strength training increases one's resting metabolic rate because muscle tissue has high energy requirements (Lamb 1985; Johnson 1986).

It has therefore been suggested that strength training has a double reducing effect (Darden 1988). A twenty-minute circuit strength training workout burns about 200 calories (Wilmore et al. 1978), which is fewer calories than a twenty-minute run utilizes. However, if as a result of regular strength training one gains two pounds of muscle, additional calories will be used twenty-four hours a day to meet the increased metabolic requirements.

Westcott (1987b) compared body composition changes for seventy-two male and female participants in a weight-loss research program. All of the subjects were advised to lose one pound per week through a combination of low-fat diet and regular exercise. The diet program was based on 20 percent fat intake, 20 percent protein intake, and 60 percent carbohydrate intake. The exercise program was based on three, thirty-minute training sessions per week for a period of eight weeks.

Twenty-two subjects performed thirty minutes of endurance exercise during each training session. The other fifty subjects performed fifteen minutes of endurance exercise and fifteen minutes of strength exercise during each training session. At the completion of the training program, the subjects who performed only endurance exercise recorded a mean fat loss of 3.0 pounds and a mean muscle loss of 0.5 pounds for a mean weight loss of 3.5 pounds. The subjects who performed both endurance exercise and strength exercise experienced a mean fat loss of 10.0 pounds and a mean muscle gain of 2.0 pounds for a mean weight loss of 8.0 pounds. The latter results actually represented a 12-pound improvement in body composition (see table 4.10). The findings of this study were similar to those in a previous investigation with twenty-four subjects (Westcott, 1985m).

Table 4.10.   Mean changes in fat, muscle, and bodyweight for subjects who did only endurance exercise and subjects who did endurance and strength exercise (N = 72).

Subjects	(N)	Fat	Muscle	Bodyweight
Endurance only	22	−3.0 lbs	−0.5 lbs	−3.5 lbs
Endurance and strength	50	−10.0 lbs	+2.0 lbs	−8.0 lbs

Summary

Dieting improves one's body composition by decreasing fat weight, but it does not increase muscle weight or resting metabolism. Aerobic exercise improves one's body composition by decreasing fat weight, but it does not increase muscle weight or resting metabolism. Strength exercise improves one's body composition by decreasing fat weight, increasing muscle weight, and increasing resting metabolism. Strength training increases caloric expenditure both during exercise and during rest, because additional muscle tissue requires additional energy supplies. Strength training is therefore an excellent means for enhancing body composition and physical appearance.

Youth Response

During the 1980s attitudes toward preadolescent strength training became much more positive (Legwold 1982; Duda 1986). Research by Clarke (1971), Westcott (1979a), Micheli (1983), Weltman et al. (1986), and others demonstrated that young boys and girls can gain strength safely. Even the American Orthopedic Society for Sports Medicine has endorsed youth strength training as long as sensible exercise guidelines are observed (see Appendix G).

Most youth fitness testing and training programs involve calisthenic exercises such as pull-ups, push-ups, and sit-ups. This is unfortunate because bodyweight exercises do not permit progressive resistance. Also, many young people are too weak to perform more than one or two repetitions in some bodyweight exercises (President's Council on Physical Fitness and Sports 1985 "National School Population Fitness Survey").

It therefore makes sense to substitute sensible strength training for bodyweight exercises. In this manner the resistance can be adjusted so that each youth can perform about ten strict repetitions per exercise, and be progressively increased upon reaching twelve repetitions.

Westcott (1988e) conducted a research study with eleven boys and girls between nine and thirteen years of age. The subjects performed twelve minutes of strength training (six Nautilus exercises) and twelve minutes of endurance training (stationary cycling) three days a week for a period of eight weeks. As shown in table 4.11, the

Table 4.11 Mean changes in muscle strength and body composition for nine- to thirteen-year-old boys and girls during eight-week exercise program (N = 11)

	Before	After	Change
Nautilus bench press	42.0 lbs.	65.6 lbs.	+23.5 lbs.
Bodyweight	137.0 lbs.	137.5 lbs	+ 0.5 lbs.
% Fat	30.0%	27.0%	− 3.0%
Fat weight	41.0 lbs.	37.0 lbs.	− 4.0 lbs.
Lean weight	95.5 lbs.	100.0 lbs.	+ 4.5 lbs.

subjects made major improvements in muscle strength and body composition. In fact, based on the ultrasound body composition assessments, the participants gained 4.5 pounds of lean weight (muscle) and lost 4.0 pounds of fat weight during the two-month training period.

Summary

Based on the results of these studies, it would appear that strength training is an effective and efficient means for improving muscle strength and body composition in preadolescent boys and girls. Because physical strength and personal appearance are important factors in peer acceptance, it is recommended that youth have the opportunity to participate in safe and supervised strength training programs.

Summary of Strength Training Research

1. *Training frequency.* Research indicates that when the weekly work output is held constant, training frequency may be a matter of individual preference. For most purposes, two or three evenly spaced training sessions per week are recommended.

2. *Training sets.*   Based on the studies reviewed, it seems that the essential stimulus for gaining strength is one high-intensity set of resistive exercise. Performing additional sets of exercise appears neither advantageous nor disadvantageous as measured by improvement in strength performance.

3. *Training repetitions.*   Research suggests that most individuals can perform eight to twelve strict repetitions with 75 percent of their maximum resistance. Most trainees will experience excellent strength results by executing eight to twelve repetitions per set of exercise.

4. *Training speed.*   Some studies revealed a specificity of training effect, while others seemed to favor slow movement speed. Because slow movement speed is characterized by greater muscle force output, it is recommended for most strength training purposes.

5. *Training time.*   Research indicates that neck extensor strength is higher in the morning than in the evening. Although one should probably train when both the energy level and strength level are highest, training time is largely a matter of personal preference.

6. *Activity order.*   One study found better results when the endurance exercise was performed before the strength exercise. However, because the performance differences were relatively small, personal objectives should be considered when designing a training protocol.

7. *Blood pressure response.*

Most of the research reviewed indicated that sensible strength training does not have an adverse affect on blood pressure in healthy adults. Some studies suggested that regular strength training may elicit positive blood pressure adaptations.

8. *Heart rate response.*

Research reveals a progressive increase in heart rate throughout a set of strength exercise. The less rest taken between successive exercises, the higher the mean heart rate response.

9. *Cardiovascular response.*

There is evidence that strength training (especially circuit strength training) may provide several positive cardiovascular effects. These include reduced resting blood pressure, improved lipoprotein and lipid profiles, increased left ventricle wall thickness, increased muscle capillarization, reduced double products, and enhanced aerobic capacity.

10. *Muscle response.*

Although strength training participants experience relatively large performance improvements during the first month of training, research indicates that this is mostly due to motor learning. That is, practice enhances neurological efficiency and enables the exerciser to use available muscle tissue more effectively. Subsequent strength gains come more slowly, but are largely the result of new muscle tissue.

11. *Body composition response.*

Research shows strength training to be an excellent means for improving body composition. Strength exercise increases lean weight (muscle) and decreases fat weight. In addition to burning calories during exercise, more muscle tissue requires more calories at rest for maintenance and building functions.

12. *Youth response.*

Research indicates that preadolescent boys and girls can improve muscle strength and body composition through sensible strength training. Because physical strength and personal appearance are important factors in peer acceptance, it is recommended that youth have the opportunity to participate in safe and supervised strength training programs.

Five

Strength Training Principles and Recommendations

People participate in strength training programs for many reasons, but predominant among these is a desire for larger and stronger muscles. Although the degree of muscular attainment is influenced by certain inherited factors such as somatotype, limb length, muscle length, angle of tendon insertion, and ratio of fast-twitch to slow-twitch muscle fibers, most people can achieve marked increases in muscle strength and hypertrophy through a systematic and progressive program of strength training. Research indicates that proper training produces the following adaptations within the muscles: a higher concentration of contractile proteins, a greater number of myofibrils per muscle fiber, a greater number of capillaries per muscle fiber, an increased amount of connective tissue, a larger percentage of muscle fibers available for force production, and a larger capacity for intramuscular energy stores (Mathews and Fox 1976; Fleck and Kraemer 1987).

There is no question that people who have engaged in widely varying programs of strength training have experienced muscular gains. Promoters of particular systems of strength augmentation are quick to point out how many champions their programs have developed. Far less publicized is the fact that strict adherence to many of these training regimens often results in muscle injury, strength decrement, and discouragement. The truth is, regardless of the training program one follows, the probability of experiencing desirable training consequences is closely related to the number of basic training principles observed by the exerciser. Conversely, the probability of encountering undesirable training consequences is closely related to the number of basic training principles violated by the exerciser.

A well-designed strength training program should incorporate the following fundamental principles of muscle development to ensure progressive improvement in strength and to reduce the risk of tissue injury: stress adaptation, rebuilding time, near-maximum resistance, movement speed, movement range, muscle balance, and continuous breathing.

Stress Adaptation

When a muscle is stressed beyond its normal demands, it reacts in some way to that stress. If the stress is slightly greater than normal, the muscle responds positively and becomes stronger. That is, after a temporary decrease in ability following the training session, the muscle gradually builds to a higher level of strength. On the other hand, if the imposed stress is too great, the muscle reacts negatively and tissue damage may result (Friden et al. 1983; Evans 1987).

As an example, if one hoes a garden for five minutes on Monday, ten minutes on Tuesday, fifteen minutes on Wednesday, and so on, the hands will gradually become calloused and hoeing can be continued for long periods of time without skin discomfort. However, if one begins by hoeing the garden for two hours on Monday, blisters are likely to develop and hoeing will have to be discontinued for several days until the skin heals. The phenomenon that occurs beneath the skin is actually quite similar.

The muscles adapt to the stress of a strength training session in some manner. If the intensity of the workout is increased gradually, the muscles respond positively and gain strength. However, if the intensity of the workout is increased abruptly, the muscles react negatively and tissue damage may occur.

According to the principle of stress adaptation, muscles require progressive increases in resistance to stimulate new growth and development. Although the means by which muscles achieve higher strength levels is not well understood, it is clear that too much stress can short-circuit the process and cause tissue injury. In fact, the immediate effect of strength training is some degree of muscle weak-

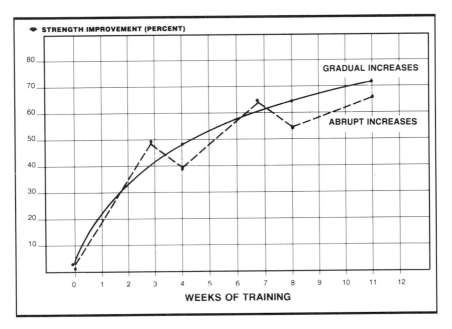

Figure 5.1 Typical progress curves for individuals who increase training stress gradually and individuals who increase training stress abruptly

ness, depending on the imposed training stress. Under proper training conditions, the muscles will be weaker but uninjured after the workout. From this posttraining low point, the muscles recover and build to slightly greater strength levels prior to the next training session.

The purpose of progressive resistance exercise is to increase muscle strength and size, and to decrease the risk of tissue injury. This purpose is best served by a long-range approach to strength development. When one is willing to progress gradually toward a strength goal, the results are generally positive and the setbacks are few. When one is in a hurry to attain strength objectives (e.g., get in top shape before football season, bench press 300 pounds before summer break), the results may still be positive but the setbacks are usually more numerous. Figure 5.1 depicts typical progress curves for patient individuals and overanxious individuals.

As discussed in chapter 4, strength performance improves more slowly after the first few weeks of training. It is therefore not advisable to increase training resistance at regular intervals, such as every

Table 5.1   Relationships for training resistance, training repetitions, and training duration

Percent of maximum resistance	Approximate number of repetitions	Approximate training duration at seven seconds per repetition
85%	6 reps.	40 secs.
80%	8 reps.	55 secs.
75%	10 reps.	70 secs.
70%	12 reps.	85 secs.
65%	14 reps.	100 secs.

two weeks. Rather, the author recommends that one remain at a given resistance until twelve repetitions can be completed in good form. When this is achieved the weightload should be increased by about 5 percent. The additional resistance will result in two or three fewer repetitions, but should permit at least eight repetitions as a new starting point. One should remain with this resistance until twelve repetitions can again be completed in good form. This process is referred to as a double progressive training program because one first adds repetitions and then adds resistance. It is a relatively conservative procedure for increasing the training stimulus, but it enables the exerciser to improve consistently with few setbacks.

Although eight to twelve repetitions is not the only effective training range, research indicates that eight repetitions corresponds to about 80 percent of one's maximum resistance and twelve repetitions corresponds to about 70 percent of one's maximum resistance (see chapter 4). Table 5.1 presents some general relationships for training resistance, training repetitions, and training duration. In the author's opinion, training between eight to twelve repetitions (70 percent to 80 percent of maximum resistance) represents a safe and effective procedure for increasing muscle strength.

The recommended 5 percent incrementation is somewhat arbitrary, but seems to work reasonably well based on experience and empirical observation. For example, if Gayle performs twelve strict repetitions with 50 pounds she should increase the resistance to 52½ pounds the next training session. She should continue to exercise with 52½ pounds until she again completes twelve repetitions, then progress to 55 pounds.

Ideally, one should improve strength performance every workout, and this is often the case during the first few weeks of training. As higher strength levels are attained, however, improvement comes more slowly, and day-to-day fluctuations become more apparent. It is therefore suggested that seasoned strength trainers not expect noticeable strength gains every workout. In fact, strength plateaus are a common occurrence that should be dealt with in a patient and positive manner (Westcott 1985a). Fortunately, not all muscle groups plateau at the same time, and one can normally see progress in some muscle groups while working on new ways to stimulate stubborn muscle groups.

Five methods for overcoming a strength plateau are: (1) changing the training exercises, (2) changing the training frequency, (3) changing the training sets, (4) changing the repetitions-resistance relationship (more repetitions with less resistance or fewer repetitions with more resistance), and (5) increasing the training intensity (breakdown training, assisted training, etc.).

The main point of progressive stress adaptation is safety. One must be careful not to progress more rapidly than the muscles' ability to recover from the training stress and rebuild to a higher strength level.

Rebuilding Time

When a muscle is stressed beyond its normal demands, a certain amount of time is required for the tissues to recover and make positive physiological adaptations (MacDougall 1985b). If the time between workouts is too short, the muscle may be unable to build to a higher level of strength before being stressed again. The cumulative effects of insufficient rebuilding time are chronically fatigued muscles that actually decrease in strength (Jones et al. 1988). Conversely, if the nontraining interval is too long, the muscles will gradually return to their original level of contractile force.

Because the length of the rest interval depends on the intensity of the work interval, more hours are required for muscle rebuilding following a hard workout than after an easy workout (Westcott 1974). Each person must experimentally determine the optimal recovery period between workouts for his or her particular training program.

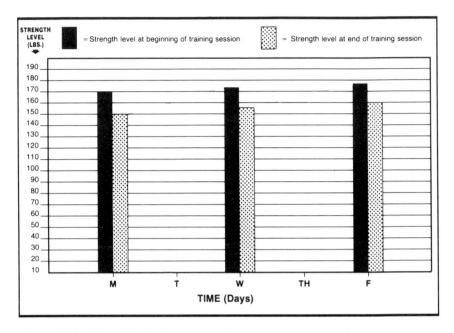

Figure 5.2 Hypothetical pattern of muscle response when recovery period is appropriate with respect to training intensity. When sufficient rest is obtained between training sessions, the muscle rebuilds to a slightly higher level of strength.

Figure 5.2 schematically illustrates that the contractile force of a muscle decreases during a training session due to the stress imposed on it, but increases to a slightly higher strength level during a recovery period of sufficient duration.

As indicated in figure 5.3 when too little rest is obtained between training sessions, the muscle is unable to build to a higher level of strength prior to the next workout. The cumulative stress of repeated training sessions without sufficient time for muscle rebuilding leads to chronic training fatigue, and the muscles actually become weaker rather than stronger.

When too much rest is taken between successive workouts, the muscle initially builds to a higher level of strength, but gradually returns to its original strength level prior to the next training session. Because the new strength level is not maintained indefinitely, it is important that the subsequent training stimulus occur near the peak of the rebuilding curve. Taking too much rest between training

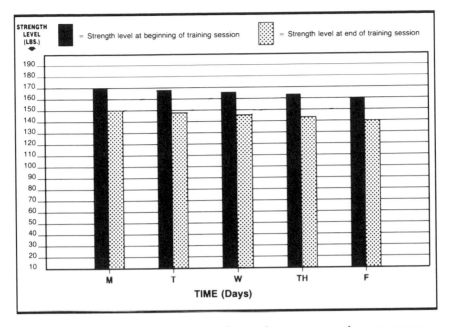

Figure 5.3 Hypothetical pattern of muscle response when recovery period is too short with respect to training intensity. When too little rest is obtained between training sessions, the muscle is unable to rebuild to a higher level of strength.

sessions may not be harmful, but the lack of strength gains can be frustrating. The consequences of an extended recovery period are illustrated schematically in figure 5.4.

Overtraining is an occupational hazard among athletes. Distance runners used to train every other day, then every day, then twice a day. The result has been moderate decreases in running times and major increases in running injuries. The body needs time to recover from the training stress and to respond to the training stimulus. This is especially true for high-intensity activities that require high levels of force production and energy utilization. Strength training and long sprints (440 yards, 880 yards) fall into this category. Persons who perform high-intensity exercise typically recover within forty-eight hours, and therefore respond well to three training sessions per week.

Some people can make continued progress with more frequent strength training sessions, while other people require three days to

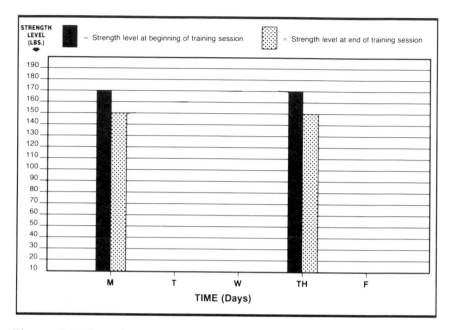

Figure 5.4 Hypothetical pattern of muscle response when recovery period is too long with respect to training intensity. When too much rest is taken between training sessions, the muscle initially rebuilds to a slightly higher level of strength, but gradually returns to its original strength level.

recuperate from hard workouts. The only way to determine one's ideal recovery time is through trial-and-error experimentation. If the training weightloads feel a little lighter than last time, then the rest period is appropriate. Ideally, one should realize some improvement in each successive workout, at least until relatively high strength levels are attained.

Training consistency is essential for optimum strength results. The person who frequently misses workouts will fail to build on the previous strength foundation and will allow the deconditioning process to begin prior to the next training session. On the other hand, when one takes workouts back to back, the muscles don't have time to regain their previous strength level, let alone become stronger.

As a basic training recommendation, most participants are advised to follow a three-day-per-week workout program. It is suggested that one exercise all of the major muscle groups each training day and rest all of the major muscle groups each nontraining day. For those who cannot commit to three training days per week, two equally-spaced exercise sessions per week may produce excellent strength results (Westcott 1986e).

Near-Maximum Resistance

There are basically two ways to apply stress to one's muscles. One may perform numerous repetitions against low resistance (e.g., jogging, cycling, rope jumping) to improve cardiovascular endurance, or one may perform few repetitions against high resistance (e.g., lifting heavy weights) to improve muscular strength and size. Each type of training stimulus produces specific results. If one's objective is to develop muscular strength and hypertrophy, the training program should focus on few repetitions with relatively heavy resistance.

The principle of near-maximum resistance is often referred to as the overload principle because strength gains are dependent upon weightloads over and above those generally encountered in one's daily activities. Research (Berger 1965; McDonagh and Davies 1984) indicates that one should train with at least 65 percent of his or her maximum weightload to obtain significant strength gains. The author therefore considers weightloads above 65 percent of maximum to constitute the category of near-maximum resistance. Although this category includes a wide range of repetitions-resistance relationships, strength training authorities generally agree that weightloads around 75 percent of maximum are highly effective for developing muscle strength and size. For most people, this corresponds to the heaviest weightload that can be lifted ten times, and is referred to as the ten-repetition maximum (10 RM) weightload (Westcott 1986l; Rhoades and Westcott 1986).

For optimum strength gains, the principle of near-maximum resistance must be applied with a high level of exercise intensity. High-intensity training means pushing one's muscles to the point where they can no longer contract concentrically. That is, until they are completely fatigued and can no longer move the resistance. This state is sometimes referred to as momentary muscle failure, because the muscles have reached their temporary functional limit.

One can conceivably reach momentary muscle failure by performing 1 repetition with 300 pounds or by doing 300 repetitions with 10 pounds. However, the former method carries a high risk of injury, and the latter method provides little stimulus for strength gain. As discussed in the previous section, 8 to 12 repetitions is a safe and effective training range for most people, as long as the resistance is sufficient to cause momentary muscle failure.

As an illustration of high-intensity training, assume that during John's last workout he completed ten repetitions with seventy-five pounds in the leg extension exercise. Today he also places seventy-five pounds on the weightstack and begins to exercise. He performs the first six repetitions slowly and with moderate effort. Although the seventh and eighth repetitions are difficult, John maintains good form and full movement range. The ninth and tenth repetitions produce considerable discomfort in his quadriceps muscles, and John can barely attain complete leg extension. He attempts another repetition, but experiences momentary muscle failure and cannot move the weight beyond the midpoint. John does not use other muscle groups, momentum, or poor form to "kick out" the final repetition. He simply squeezes the muscles in a deliberate manner until they are overcome by the resistance. If John had stopped at the completion of ten repetitions, he would have missed the added stimulus for muscle development. By continuing to exercise in good form to the limit of his contractile capacity, John achieved a high-intensity training effort.

Although this type of training is very demanding, it is occasionally desirable to work the muscles even more intensely. One method for making the exercise set even more stressful is to reduce the weightload at the point of momentary muscle failure and force out a few more repetitions with a lighter resistance. This is referred to as breakdown training.

For example, let's assume that John has 100 available muscle fibers, and that each muscle fiber exerts one pound of force. In order to lift seventy-five pounds in the leg extension, John requires 75 contracting muscle fibers. As John continues to exercise, some muscle fibers fatigue and can no longer exert force. After ten repetitions 26 muscle fibers are fatigued, and John cannot lift the seventy-five pound weightload. If he immediately reduces the resistance by ten pounds, he may be able to complete two or three more repetitions and fatigue another 10 muscles fibers. By so doing, he has hypothetically exhausted 36 of the 100 muscle fibers at the completion of the extended exercise set during which he has experienced muscle failure twice.

This is a painful means of training, but it may actually provide a more intense stimulus than performing three sets of ten repetitions with the same weightload. Resting between sets permits the fatigued fibers to recover. Because each set is discontinued when seventy-five pounds can no longer be lifted, only about 26 of the 100 muscle fibers hypothetically reach exhaustion even though several sets are performed.

For most purposes, one set of exercise that produces momentary muscle failure between eight and twelve repetitions is sufficient training stimulus for strength development (Westcott 1987b; Westcott 1988e; Westcott et al. 1989). However, when greater muscle stimulus is desired, breakdown training offers a controlled means of reaching deeper into one's strength reserves. Assisted training is another means for achieving the same objective by receiving help from a training partner during the last few repetitions. That is, the training partner lifts a small percentage of the resistance so that the exerciser can complete two or three additional repetitions and thereby fatigue more muscle fibers.

Movement Speed

When training with weights, it is important to raise and lower the weightload in a slow and controlled manner to ensure consistent application of force throughout the exercise movement. Such movements provide the muscles with more or less steady stress during both the lifting phase (concentric contraction) and the lowering phase (eccentric contraction).

Experiments with force plates have revealed that lifting movements performed at a moderate speed require a relatively even application of muscular force. On the other hand, executing fast repetitions with a barbell or dumbbell is equivalent to throwing the weight. It seems that fast movements demand excessive muscular force at the beginning of the lift, but practically no muscle force is necessary during the midrange of the lift. Tests have demonstrated that during explosive lifting movements, the exerciser is actually lifted by the weights. In fact, electronic traces of a quick press with a 60-pound barbell show a range of forces from over 100 pounds at the start of the lift to less than zero during the middle part of the lift (Wolf 1981).

There can be little doubt that rapidly accelerating and decelerating a weightload subjects the muscles to widely varying levels of stress. Consequently, explosive strength training movements carry a higher risk of tissue injury.

It should also be recalled that near-maximum resistance is a key to strength development. As the speed of movement increases, however, the weightload must necessarily be reduced unless assisting muscles are utilized. Therefore, fast lifting movements may be less effective for strength development. Consider the following six reasons for using slow strength training technique.

More Muscle Tension

Slow strength training produces a longer period of continuous muscle tension. A slow lifting movement provides a longer period of muscle tension during the concentric contraction, and a slow lowering movement provides a longer period of muscle tension during the eccentric contraction.

For example, a fast-paced, one-second-up and one-second-down training cadence requires only twenty seconds of continuous muscle tension to complete ten repetitions. On the other hand, a slow-paced, two-second-up, one-second-pause, and four-second-down training cadence requires seventy seconds of continuous muscle tension to complete ten repetitions. Given the same weightload, both methods accomplish the same amount of work. However, the slower technique involves more muscle tension, and muscle tension is important for strength development.

More Muscle Force

When evaluated isokinetically, maximum strength tests invariably reveal that more muscle force is produced at slower movement speeds than at faster movement speeds. As illustrated in figure 5.5, as the movement speed increases the maximum force output decreases. That is, isokinetic movements of 60 degrees per second produce more muscle force than isokinetic movements of 120 degrees per second, and isokinetic movements of 120 degrees per second pro-

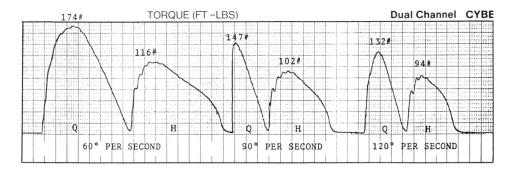

Figure 5.5 Isokinetic assessment of muscle force production at various movement speeds

duce more muscle force than isokinetic movements at 180 degrees per second. Because muscle force output is greater at slower movement speeds, it would appear that slow strength training is more effective than fast strength training for muscle development (Clarke and Manning 1985).

More Muscle Fibers

Muscle force can be increased by activating more muscle fibers, speeding up the firing rate, or both. Because the firing rate at slow speeds does not exceed the firing rate at fast speeds, the greater muscle force produced at slow speeds is apparently due to greater recruitment of muscle fibers. Research indicates that forceful contractions utilize both fast-twitch and slow-twitch muscle fibers (Lesmes et al. 1983). It therefore appears that slow strength training provides more time to activate both muscle fiber types, resulting in greater force production.

More Muscle Power

Power is the product of force times speed. Power can therefore be enhanced by increasing muscle force, movement speed, or both. This may be more difficult than it appears, because there is an optimum combination of force and speed necessary for maximum power output. The author therefore recommends that one perform high-intensity strength training to improve muscle force and high-quality

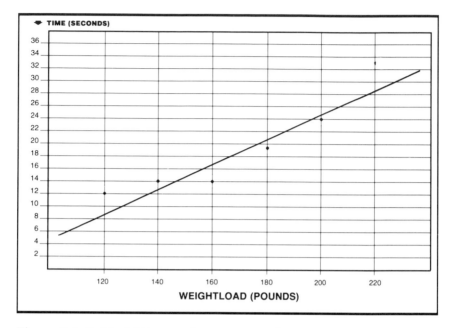

Figure 5.6 Subjects' time-resistance curve for executing ten strict repetitions in the bench press exercise. Note that as the weightload increases, the repetitions are necessarily performed more slowly, even though the subject is exercising as fast as control allows.

skill training to improve movement speed. Trying to develop both components in a single workout may be counterproductive.

As shown in figure 5.6, it takes longer to perform ten strict repetitions with a heavy resistance than with a light resistance. Because near-maximum resistance is essential for muscle force development, it is recommended that one train with relatively heavy weightloads and relatively slow speeds.

Less Tissue Trauma

Speed is an essential ingredient in any power event. However, most power events are performed with bodyweight (e.g., long jump, high jump) or with relatively light implements (e.g., shot, discus). Power events performed with heavy resistance (e.g., clean and jerk) place great stress on joint structures, thereby increasing the risk of tissue trauma.

The faster one accelerates an object, the greater the stress on the involved tendons, ligaments, and muscle fascia. Slow lifting movements accomplish the same amount of work as fast lifting movements. However, slow strength training provides a more consistent application of muscle tension and muscle force, thereby reducing tissue trauma and injury potential. For this reason alone, slow strength training technique should be given careful consideration.

Less Momentum

Momentum plays a part in virtually all weight-training exercises. The faster the lifting movement, the greater the momentum. This is an important consideration because as the momentum component increases, the muscle component decreases.

There are many means for generating momentum. The most common technique involves the use of assisting muscle groups to begin the lifting movement (e.g., using the hip extensor muscles to initiate barbell curls). Although heavier weightloads can be utilized in this manner, the target muscle group may actually receive less training stimulus due to the momentum factor.

Another example of momentum assisted weight training is bouncing the barbell off the chest during the bench press exercise. In addition to the high injury potential, this careless use of momentum reduces the training effect on the target muscle groups.

While momentum certainly has its place in sporting events, it should probably play a minor role in strength training programs. Momentum-assisted weight training gives the appearance of greater muscle strength, but generally decreases demands on the target muscles and increases stress on the joint structures.

Based on these six arguments for slow strength training technique and on the research results presented in chapter 4, it is recommended that lifting movements be performed at about sixty degrees per second. This corresponds to about two seconds for most strength training movements.

Because lowering movements are easier due to gravity and muscle friction, it is suggested that the lowering phase be performed even more slowly. As a rule of thumb, four seconds provides a safe and effective eccentric contraction. The author recommends a two-second lifting movement, a one-second pause, and a four-second lowering movement for most strength training exercises. In this manner, ten repetitions can be completed in about seventy seconds.

Movement Range

Almost everyone agrees that it is important to exercise through a full range of movement to strengthen the muscles at all joint positions and to maintain joint flexibility.

The author emphasizes the fully-contracted position of each exercise movement. With respect to strength, a fully-contracted muscle is characterized by near-maximum contact between the actin and myosin filaments. A momentary isometric contraction in the fully-shortened position may therefore enhance the strength stimulus.

With respect to flexibility, whenever one muscle group is fully contracted, the opposite muscle group is fully stretched. For example, as one performs a triceps exercise, the triceps muscles shorten and the biceps muscles lengthen. At the end point of the exercise, the triceps muscles are in a completely contracted position and the biceps muscles are in a fully stretched position. Conversely, as one performs a biceps exercise, the biceps muscles shorten and the triceps muscles lengthen. At the end point of the exercise, the biceps muscles are in a completely contracted position and the triceps muscles are in a fully stretched position.

Exercise range should be taken into consideration when selecting exercise movements, because the distance over which a muscle moves a resistance is proportional to the amount of work done:

$$\text{Work} = \text{Force} \times \text{Distance}$$

For example, chin-ups performed with a narrow, palms-in grip provide a greater movement range than chin-ups performed with a wide, palms-out grip. Because a longer movement range requires a longer muscle contraction, it is generally more effective for strength development.

It is important to use an appropriate exercise resistance. For example, if John uses 100 pounds he can achieve full knee extension for ten repetitions in the leg extension exercise. If John uses 120 pounds, he can achieve full knee extension for only four repetitions. It is probably more beneficial for John to train with full muscle contractions at 100 pounds and develop strength throughout the entire movement range.

It is recommended that whenever possible, exercises be performed slowly and smoothly through a complete range of movement. One should not force the muscles into painful positions, but should attempt to attain a reasonably stretched position and a fully contracted position on each repetition. When complete muscle contraction cannot be attained, breakdown training or assisted training may enable the exerciser to perform two or three additional repetitions through a full range of movement.

Muscle Balance

Weight training programs should be designed to promote strength development in all of the major muscle groups. Emphasizing certain muscle groups can produce muscle imbalance which may, in time, lead to muscle injury. For example, football players typically train their quadriceps muscles harder than their hamstring muscles. This often results in a relatively strong quadriceps group and a relatively weak hamstrings group that becomes highly susceptible to injury (Fleck and Falkel 1986; Baratta et al. 1988).

Whenever a muscle group is disproportionately stronger than its antagonist, the latter is predisposed to injury. This is not to say that paired muscle groups should be trained to exactly equal strength. For example, the quadriceps muscles are stronger than the hamstring muscles at the knee joint (knee extension versus knee flexion), but the hamstring muscles are stronger than the quadriceps muscles at the hip joint (hip extension versus hip flexion). Consequently, one would normally use more resistance in knee extension than knee flexion and in hip extension than hip flexion.

The important point is that the muscle groups should not be trained in isolation. If the muscles on one side of a joint are worked, then the muscles on the opposite side of the joint should likewise be worked, even though the weightloads may not be identical.

The problem of maintaining desirable muscle balance can be simplified by training all of the major muscle groups, including the quadriceps, hamstrings, hip adductors, hip abductors, low back, abdominals, obliques, pectoralis, upper back, deltoids, biceps, triceps, neck flexors, and neck extensors. Furthermore, one should not work the wrist extensors without also training the wrist flexors or the calf muscles apart from the shin muscles (see chapter 7).

The principle of muscle balance is a necessary counterpart to the concept of training specificity. To many people, training specificity means training only those muscle groups that are prime movers for a particular event. For example, a thrower may perform a variety of triceps exercises to improve his shot put performance. However, unless the triceps exercises are balanced with biceps exercises, he will increase the risk of overuse injuries. It appears that overly specialized training has been at least partially responsible for numerous injuries to muscle and connective tissue.

The concept of training specificity may be applied to energy systems. For example, sprinters should spend the majority of their training time performing high-intensity, anaerobic running exercise. Conversely, distance runners should spend the majority of their training time performing low-intensity, aerobic running exercise.

It is also suggested that the concept of training specificity be applied to sports skills. For example, the high jump is a very complex athletic event. Although high jumpers should certainly execute a variety of jumping drills, it is recommended that their technique practice emphasize full speed jumps with the crossbar at challenging heights.

Regardless of one's performance objectives, a sound strength training program should include exercises for all of the major muscle groups. Balanced development of one's musculature sets a firm foundation for further improvement and minimizes the risk of overuse injuries.

Continuous Breathing

Before experimenting with various strength training exercises, one should understand something about proper breathing during forceful muscular contraction. Taking a deep breath and holding it while straining to complete a repetition is a dangerous practice. The internal pressure created by breath holding coupled with the external pressure of tightly contracted muscles may be sufficient to limit blood flow and cause a feeling of lightheadedness.

Perhaps more important, the increased pressure in the chest area that results from holding the breath during a strenuous lifting movement can interfere with venous blood return to the heart and significantly elevate blood pressure. This undesirable reaction is known as the Valsalva response. Consequently, the breath should never be held for a prolonged period of time when exercising with weights.

From a physiological standpoint, the best system of breathing requires the exerciser to inhale during the lowering movement (eccentric contraction) and to exhale during the lifting movement (concentric contraction). In this manner, the air pressure decreases as the muscular pressure increases and vice versa.

Most exercisers develop a breathing pattern that suits their particular training style without jeopardizing blood flow or restricting their oxygen supply. As long as one breathes regularly and does not hold the breath for more than a moment, problems should not be encountered.

Summary of Strength Training Principles and Recommendations

Strength training should not be a hit-or-miss activity. Proper program design is a critical factor in any strength training endeavor. By applying the seven principles presented in this chapter, one can experience safe and successful strength training that increases muscle fitness and reduces the risk of injury.

1.	*Stress adaptation.*	Because physiological adaptations in muscle tissue occur slowly, resistance should not be increased abruptly. As a rule of thumb, one should increase the weightload by 5 percent when twelve repetitions can be completed in proper form.
2.	*Rebuilding time.*	Because intense muscle training usually requires forty-eight hours recovery and rebuilding time, one should generally schedule three nonconsecutive workout days per week.

3. *Near-maximum resistance.*   For optimum strength gains, one should typically use a resistance heavy enough to cause momentary muscle failure within eight to twelve strict exercise repetitions.

4. *Movement speed.*   To increase muscle tension and to decrease the risk of injury, strength training exercises should be performed slowly. Generally speaking, the lifting movement should take about two seconds and the lowering movement should take about four seconds.

5. *Movement range.*   For maximum muscle benefit each exercise should be performed through a full range of movement, with a momentary pause in the completely contracted position.

6. *Muscle balance.*   At least one exercise should be performed for each of the major muscle groups. These include the quadriceps, hamstrings, hip abductors, hip adductors, low back, abdominals, obliques, pectoralis, upper back, deltoids, biceps, triceps, neck extensors, and neck flexors.

7. *Continuous breathing.*   It is essential to breathe continuously during strength exercise. For best results, one should inhale during eccentric contractions and exhale during concentric contractions.

Six

Strength Training Design and Management

There are many factors that should be considered when designing a strength fitness facility. Likewise, there are important training and management decisions that affect the day-to-day fitness operation. This chapter presents some of these concerns and offers some practical suggestions for successful strength training design and management.

Safety Considerations

Equipment

The first safety consideration is equipment. It is imperative to purchase quality exercise equipment and to keep the equipment in excellent working condition. Every piece of strength training equipment should be periodically inspected for structural weaknesses and mechanical shortcomings. Large facilities may be well-advised to consider preventive maintenance contracts with reputable equipment repair companies. As a general guideline, strength training equipment should undergo preventive maintenance overhauls every three months. Special attention should be given to welded areas; supportive structures; and moving parts such as cables, chains, pulleys, and sprockets.

Unsafe or questionable equipment should be taken out of service and, if possible, removed from the facility until it is repaired. Although most free weights are quite durable, cracked dumbbells, barbell plates, and collars should be quickly replaced.

Space

The second safety consideration is space. Few things present a greater safety threat than too many people in too little space. Many fitness centers overcrowd their training rooms, making it difficult to move around without interfering with other exercisers.

As a rule of thumb, it is not advisable to place more than fifteen strength machines in 1,000 square feet of training space. Because barbells and dumbbells can be used in almost unrestricted movement patterns, free-weight stations should have even larger buffer zones.

In high-use facilities, it is a good idea to establish participant traffic patterns to enhance the training experience and reduce the accident potential. For example, if all exercisers move down the lines of equipment in order from larger to smaller muscle groups, there should be little confusion.

If stretching is encouraged, there should be ample space for participants to perform flexibility exercises. Stretching should not be permitted between exercise stations or in walkways. Empirical evidence suggests that space sensitivity leads to better training sessions and greater member satisfaction, as well as a safer exercise facility.

Spotters

The third safety consideration is the use of spotters for certain barbell exercises, such as squats and bench presses. In each of these exercises, inability to raise the barbell from the bottom position has potentially harmful consequences. It is therefore advisable to incorporate a spotter when performing these and other exercises. The spotter should give the exerciser plenty of space to perform the lifting movement, but be ready to help the moment assistance is required.

More specifically, when spotting the bench press exercise, the spotter may assist in lifting the barbell from the standards and returning the barbell to the standards. If assistance is needed to raise the barbell, the spotter should grasp the barbell firmly and apply lifting force with the legs as well as the arms. When spotting the squat, the spotter should stand behind the exerciser and move up and down in tandem. If the upward movement stalls out, the spotter should wrap his arms around the exerciser's chest and help him to the standing position. Needless to say, the spotter uses his leg muscles for the majority of force production.

Training Technique

The fourth, and perhaps most important safety consideration, is training technique. Undoubtedly, improper exercise technique is responsible for more strength training injuries than all other causes combined. Most training injuries result from too much weight, too much speed, or too little support.

When too much weight is used for the target muscles to handle, additional muscle groups are utilized to produce momentum. Momentum-assisted weight lifting is a dangerous procedure because it subjects the muscles, tendons, and connective tissue to high stress levels.

Too much speed has a similar effect on soft tissue and joint structures. Fast exercise speeds tend to produce excessive stress at the beginning and end of each lifting movement, thereby increasing the risk of injury.

Too little support is a frequent cause of low back injuries, particularly when performing overhead pressing exercises. As illustrated in figure 6.1, such movements tend to force an arched back position with associated stress to the low back area.

For the sake of safety, it is not advisable to perform exercises with too much weight, too much speed, or too little support. Generally speaking, the training weightload should permit at least eight good repetitions. For most people, eight repetitions corresponds to about 80 percent of their maximum weightload, which represents a relatively safe training effort.

Although control is the major objective, movement speeds of about sixty degrees per second provide a safe and effective training stimulus. This corresponds to about two seconds per lifting movement for most strength training exercises.

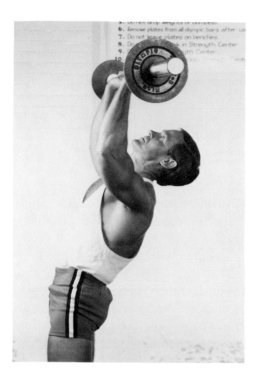

Figure 6.1 Unsupported overhead press

Unsupported exercises that place undue stress on the lower back should be replaced with safer strength training exercises. For example, by performing overhead pressing exercises on an incline bench one maintains support behind the back and reduces stress to the low back muscles (see figure 6.2).

Equipment Characteristics

Resistance Factors

The key to strength development is progressive resistance. That is, to gain more strength one must use more resistance. Because bodyweight exercises such as push-ups and sit-ups use progressive repetitions rather than progressive resistance, they are not very effective for building muscle strength.

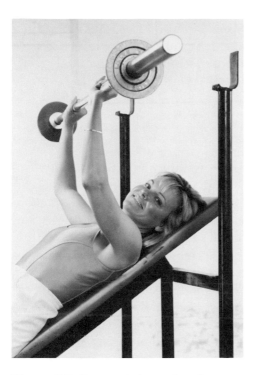

Figure 6.2 Supported overhead press

Progressive resistance can be provided in many forms, including weights, electrical resistance, air pressure, and hydraulic pressure. Although the type of resistance may be different, the strength training principles are exactly the same. The results may vary, however, based on the type of equipment utilized.

For example, hydraulic equipment provides isokinetic resistance. In isokinetic training the movement speed is constant, and the amount of force one produces determines the amount of resistance one receives. The more force one applies the more resistance one encounters, and the less force one applies the less resistance one encounters. Depending on the equipment, isokinetic exercise may offer resistance during both concentric and eccentric contractions, or only during concentric contractions.

Exercises performed with weights, either free weights or weightstack machines, provide isotonic resistance that may be constant or variable. In isotonic training, the amount of resistance one uses determines the amount of force one produces. The more resistance one uses the more force one must apply, and the less resistance one uses the less force one must apply. Isotonic training offers resistance during both the concentric and eccentric phase of the exercise movement.

Free Weights and Weightstack Machines

Although the majority of strength training participants use isotonic exercises, some prefer free weights while others prefer weightstack machines. Perhaps the major advantages of free weights are freedom of movement with largely unrestricted exercise patterns, and the incorporation of stabilizer muscles for balance and coordination. On the other hand, machine exercises may have certain advantages with regards to muscle isolation and variable resistance.

Let's compare a common free-weight exercise, dumbbell flies, and a representative machine exercise, the ten-degree chest, with respect to four strength training factors. Both exercises are intended to strengthen the pectoralis major and anterior deltoid muscles.

Supportive Structure

Supportive structure is important for safety purposes, particularly with regard to the lower back. As illustrated in figure 6.3 and 6.4, both dumbbell flies and the ten-degree chest exercise provide support for the lower back. Some exercisers place their feet on the bench to flatten the lower back while others keep their feet on the floor to enhance stability. In either case, it is essential to keep the hips on the bench throughout the exercise.

Rotary Movement

Basically, an exercise movement is either linear (straight) or rotary (curved). Generally speaking, linear movements involve two or more joint actions whereas rotary movements involve a single joint action. Consequently, rotary movements are advantageous for isolating target muscle groups. Both dumbbell flies and the ten-degree chest exercise produce rotary movement of the arms about the shoulder axes. This action, horizontal shoulder flexion, emphasizes the pectoralis major and anterior deltoid muscles (see figures 6.3 and 6.4).

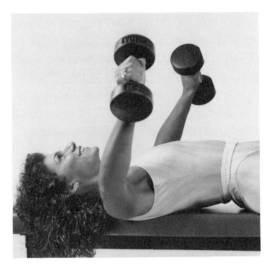

Figure 6.3 Supported dumbbell fly

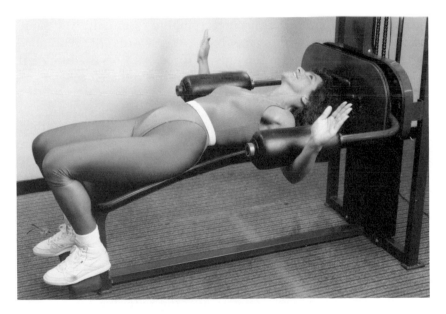

Figure 6.4 Supported ten-degree chest exercise

Direct Resistance

Direct resistance is another means for isolating target muscle groups. Because dumbbell flies require the exerciser to grip the handles, the forearm and arm muscles are actively involved in this exercise. Should these muscle groups fatigue first, the exercise must be terminated even though the pectoralis major and anterior deltoid muscles have not been worked to capacity. Conversely, the ten-degree chest exercise places the resistance pads directly against the arms, to which the target muscles attach. With direct resistance, the forearm and arm muscles are bypassed, and the exercise may be continued until the pectoralis major and anterior deltoid muscle are fatigued.

Variable Resistance

Another aspect of free-weight training that should be considered is leverage changes. Due to leverage factors the first phase of the dumbbell fly is a relatively weak muscle position, and the last phase of the dumbbell fly is a relatively strong muscle position. Unfortunately, the dumbbell resistance remains essentially the same throughout the exercise movement. In other words, the resistance force is not well-matched to the muscle force. As a result, dumbbell flies have a rather high injury potential and a rather low strength building potential.

The ten-degree chest machine attempts to compensate for the leverage changes by means of a counter leverage system. As illustrated in figure 6.5, an oval cam and chain arrangement automatically changes the resistance throughout the movement range. Because the first phase of the ten-degree chest exercise is a relatively weak muscle position, the cam provides a relatively low resistance. Because the last phase of the ten-degree chest exercise is a relatively strong muscle position, the cam provides a relatively high resistance. Unlike dumbbell flies, the resistive force is reasonably well-matched to the muscle force throughout the exercise movement. Due to variable resistance, the ten-degree chest exercise has a rather low injury potential and a rather high strength building potential.

Whether training with free weights or weightstack machines, the visual feedback serves as an excellent source of reinforcement. Most people like to see tangible evidence of their exercise efforts and the addition of weight plates clearly indicates performance progress.

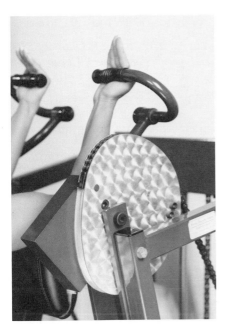

Figure 6.5 Oval cam and chain

Table 6.1 provides comparative information on several types of popular strength training equipment. Although they may differ somewhat in safety, effectiveness, efficiency, and expense, they are all useful for increasing muscle strength as long as the basic training principles are followed. Regardless of the equipment utilized, injury prevention and strength development are directly related to the basic training recommendations presented in chapter 5.

Equipment Maintenance

One of the most important aspects of a successful strength training facility is well-maintained equipment. Few things are more disappointing to participants than an out-of-order sign on a piece of equipment. Equipment maintenance is not synonomous with equipment repair. The major objective of equipment maintenance is to stop trouble before it starts.

Table 6.1   Comparative chart of various types of strength training equipment

Features	Barbell Type	Universal gym type	Nautilus type	Hydraulic type	Compressed air type	Computerized type
Safety features	No	Yes	Yes	Yes	Yes	Yes
Durability	Yes	Yes	Yes	Yes	Yes	Too new to determine
Concentric contractions	Yes	Yes	Yes	Yes	Yes	Yes
Eccentric contractions	Yes	Yes	Yes	No	Yes	Some yes Some no
Static contractions	Yes	Yes	Yes	No	Yes	Some yes Some no
Rotary movement (all major muscles)	No	Some yes Some no	Yes	Yes	Yes	No
Direct resistance (all major muscles)	No	Some yes Some no	Yes	Yes	Yes	No
Variable resistance (all major muscles)	No	No	Yes	Yes	Yes	Yes
Observable resistance	Yes	Yes	Yes	No	No	No

Preventive maintenance makes a significant difference in both equipment function and equipment repair. Properly maintained equipment works better and breaks down less often.

Barbell and dumbbell maintenance is relatively simple, generally requiring nothing more than safety checks and an occasional coating of light oil to prevent corrosion. Benches should be routinely inspected for loose bolts, cracks and other weaknesses. Small punctures in the upholstery should be immediately repaired with a sealing substance, and ripped covering should be replaced. It is wise to have additional bench pads on hand so that the damaged pad can be re-covered without putting the bench out of service for more than a few minutes.

Although most strength training machines are well-constructed and reasonably durable, their moving parts require daily inspection and care. Cables must be checked for wear, and replaced long before there is any chance of breaking. Chains and sprockets should be observed for possible problems and lubricated according to the manufacturer's specifications.

Perhaps most critical for smooth machine function are sparkling clean guiderods upon which the weightstacks travel. If the guiderods are not smooth frictional forces will be increased, making it harder to raise the weightstack and easier to lower the weightstack. This is counter-productive because our muscles are weaker in the lifting movement (concentric contraction) and stronger in the lowering movement (eccentric contraction). The guiderods should be wiped down on a daily basis with an appropriate cleaning/lubricating spray. It is important to remove as much residue as possible to reduce dust attraction.

For purposes of sanitation as well as protection, it is a good idea to place a spray bottle of disinfectant/cleanser solution and a hand towel at every machine. Each participant should wipe down the upholstery after completing the exercise. By so doing the upholstery lasts longer, looks better, and smells better. In addition, members have the opportunity to demonstrate courtesy to each other and responsibility for the equipment.

To reduce the risk of machine breakdown it is advisable to schedule equipment overhauls every three months. Many strength training facilities have professional preventive maintenance contracts to assure that their equipment remains in excellent condition and that worn parts are replaced before they become troublesome.

It is also a wise investment to have additional parts in stock, particularly extra pads, weightstack pins, saddleweights, seat belts, and upholstery. In fact, it is helpful to use velcro-secured upholstery coverings over the elbow and knee pressure areas. In this manner, the upholstery coverings can be easily replaced without removing the pads and interrupting equipment use.

There comes a time in the life of all equipment when some aesthetic attention is necessary. Generally, this type of equipment maintenance can be conducted on a yearly basis, and includes touch-up painting on machine frames, repainting weightstacks, and refelting saddle plates.

In like manner, once a year is not too often to make minor changes in the strength training facility. These include touch-up painting on walls and doors, new wall hangings, plant rearrangement, equipment repositioning, workout card revision, and other adjustments to enhance the training environment.

Equipment maintenance is an ongoing process that extends far beyond repair service. Prevention is the key to equipment that functions properly, and planning is the key to equipment that is used properly.

Facility Design

The design of the strength training facility has a lot to do with the utilization of the strength training facility. The easier it is for members to use the exercise facility, the greater the level of participation and the higher the level of satisfaction.

Ease of utilization is not the same as free use of the exercise area. Unstructured and unsupervised exercise facilities may be acceptable under certain circumstances, but they are not conducive to safe, effective, and efficient strength training with large groups of participants.

Poorly designed and under-managed training facilities are characterized by a "me first" attitude that often leads to a few dominant exercisers and a lot of frustrated members. Lack of order, in either equipment layout or training procedures, significantly reduces the opportunity for most participants to experience a satisfactory training session.

The exercise area should be designed in accordance with the basic strength training recommendations. Generally speaking, exercisers should be able to utilize the equipment in an orderly manner with minimum delay between exercise stations. In addition, each participant should have easy access to competent instructors, personal workout cards, warm-up/cool down areas, cold drinking water, and nearby locker room facilities.

Table 6.2 Sample exercises that work the major muscle groups in order from larger to smaller

Exercise Machines	Muscle Group
Leg extension	Quadriceps muscles
Leg curl	Hamstrings muscles
Hip adductor	Hip adductor muscles
Hip abductor	Hip abductor muscles
Low back	Low back muscles
Abdominal	Abdominal muscles
Rotary torso	Oblique muscles
10-degree chest	Pectoralis muscles
Super pullover	Upper back muscles
Lateral raise	Deltoid muscles
Biceps curl	Biceps muscles
Triceps extension	Triceps muscles
Neck flexion	Neck flexor muscles
Neck extension	Neck extensor muscles

Equipment Layout

Let's begin with the equipment layout. If space permits, it is advisable to place the exercise machines in a line that addresses all of the major muscle groups. For example, table 6.2 presents fourteen sample exercises that work the major muscle groups in order from larger to smaller.

By arranging the equipment in this manner, each exerciser experiences a comprehensive training session, working opposite muscle groups in sequence to assure balanced muscular development. Because the larger muscles use more energy, it makes sense to exercise these groups first and then proceed to the smaller muscle groups. With everyone progressing from machine to machine in the same direction, there should be few problems with traffic flow or movement patterns between stations.

Training Policy

The next step to consider is a facility training policy. In some facilities participants perform one set of each exercise as they move down a line of machines designed to work all of the major muscle groups. An advantage of this system is that the members know what to expect when they come for a workout. They are not worried about long delays because someone is dominating a particular exercise station. They are not concerned that someone will jump on the next machine just before they are ready to use it. Instead, they know that the other participants are moving in the same direction and taking about the same amount of time for each exercise as themselves.

Most members appreciate structured exercise facilities that foster conformity to the basic training guidelines. Consider the confusion and chaos that would result if every person in an aerobic dance class moved in a different direction. The same logic applies to a well-designed and well-managed strength training facility. It is therefore advisable to promote orderly exercise programs that enable participants to train in an efficient, productive, and problem-free manner.

Educational Emphasis

Perhaps the least understood aspect of physical fitness is the area of strength training. Bodybuilders train one way, weightlifters train another way, and football players train a different way. Free-weight users train in a different manner than machine exercisers, and every equipment manufacturer seems to advocate a specialized training technique. Most training facilities have their own method for maximum muscle development, and there is little consensus among strength experts regarding the right way to strength train. Even fitness books and strength magazines show little agreement on the best approach to muscle development.

For these reasons, it is important to place a strong emphasis on member education. Member education requires competent instruction in both general strength training principles and specific strength training practices at the facility.

Member education is an investment that takes a considerable amount of time and materials, but the dividends make it well worth the effort. The dividends include motivated members who are knowledgeable about strength exercise, who practice sensible strength training, and who attain high levels of strength fitness. These members generally take great satisfaction in their exercise achievements, and frequently encourage their family, friends, and co-workers to start a strength training program. In a sense, they become fellow educators and motivators in the area of strength fitness.

Member education may include the distribution of sound strength training books, articles, newsletters, and manuals to program participants. It may also involve strength training bulletin boards, computerized message boards, posters, pictures, and wall signs. Some strength training facilities have found strength training slide presentations to be an excellent means for participant education and member orientation.

Member Orientation

The first step to member education is an informative orientation session for every new member. As an example, consider the member orientation program at one strength fitness facility.

Step 1: Prior to training in the Strength Fitness Center, every new member must attend the strength training orientation program offered every morning and evening, Monday through Friday.

Step 2: Upon arrival the new member meets the orientation director and views two colorful slide presentations. The first is a fifteen-minute overview of strength training benefits. The second is a fifteen-minute summary of strength training guidelines.

Step 3: The new member receives a basic strength training book and a participant policy manual.

Step 4: The new member is given a body composition assessment to determine starting points in terms of percent fat, fat weight, and lean weight. A retest is scheduled for two months to observe body composition changes as a result of the exercise program. It is explained that most previously sedentary individuals lose fat weight and gain muscle weight when they follow the training recommendations.

Step 5: After answering any questions, the new member is scheduled for the first of several hands-on training sessions in the Strength Fitness Center.

Step 6:   The new member works one-on-one with an instructor for thirty minutes of training on six exercise machines, then schedules a second training session.

Step 7:   The new member works one-on-one with an instructor for thirty minutes of training on six more exercise machines, then schedules a third training session.

Step 8:   This procedure is repeated until the new member has demonstrated proper performance on all of the strength training equipment.

Step 9:   At the two-month body composition retest, the new member gives a written evaluation of the orientation program. At the same time, the orientation director answers any questions, checks the workout sheets, and makes appropriate changes to the training program. The new member is then scheduled for a one-on-one high-intensity workout with an instructor.

Step 10:   The new member experiences a high-intensity training session and is encouraged to schedule additional supervised workouts as desired.

Although somewhat costly in terms of time and materials, the strength training orientation program provides a progressive introductory experience for new members. The emphasis on member education and member supervision seems well worth the effort when it comes to member satisfaction. There appears to be a positive relationship between strength training instruction and strength training results. Good instruction fosters good results, and good results are essential for member motivation.

Member Motivation

Strength training participants expect certain things to happen as a result of their exercise efforts. In general, most members want to look better, feel better, and function better. In specific, many members expect to add muscle weight and lose fat weight. Almost everyone involved in strength training anticipates at least moderate strength gains.

Success is closely related to motivation. People tend to pursue those activities that bring success, but typically discontinue those activities that do not bring success. It is therefore important for new members to observe reasonable progress toward their strength training goals.

There are several things that instructors can do to enhance members' training motivation. These include positive reinforcement, fitness testing, self-recording, supervised training, and role modeling.

Positive Reinforcement

Positive reinforcement is a largely misunderstood concept. Although saying "Good job, John" or "Nice effort, Mary" is a form of positive reinforcement, it has limited motivational value.

Consider two categories of positive reinforcement that seem to have a greater impact on participant behavior. The first is specific positive reinforcement, and refers to the information content of a compliment. That is, telling members what is good about their performance.

For example, if an instructor says, "Good job, John, you are exercising through your full range of motion," John is more likely to continue performing full range movements. In addition to serving as meaningful reinforcement, specific comments provide useful instruction to the exerciser and to everyone who overhears.

The second category is general positive reinforcement, and refers to the attitude of the staff and the atmosphere of the facility. Most members have a sixth sense that tells them whether they are in a user-friendly environment or a user-unfriendly environment. The former is usually staffed by instructors who call members by name, who check form and progress, and who act positively and professionally whenever they are on duty.

It is characterized by a clean, well-structured facility that fosters trouble-free utilization. That means ample equipment, smooth traffic flow, good supervision, and an emphasis on member courtesy. It includes spray bottles and towels on the machines, easy-to-read instructional charts, a convenient workout card system, easy room access, cold water dispensers, informative bulletin boards, and enthusiastic instructors. It also features a friendly and progressive new member orientation program.

Fitness Testing

Fitness testing is perhaps the best means of demonstrating physical improvement to program participants. Although some exercise adaptations are obvious, others are not. For example, many people pursue strength training to enhance their physical appearance. Unfortunately, they often equate physical appearance with bodyweight. As it is not uncommon to train for two months without any change in bodyweight, some people become discouraged and discontinue their programs.

However, if these same participants had received body composition assessments they may have realized a three-pound gain in muscle weight and a three-pound loss in fat weight. What appeared to be wasted effort may have actually produced a six-pound change in body composition, with related improvements in physical capacity and metabolic function. It is therefore recommended that accurate body composition assessments be available to all strength training participants.

Another fitness parameter that should be evaluated for program members is muscle strength. It may be useful to consider the following criteria when selecting a test for muscle strength: (1) low risk of injury; (2) targets a major muscle group involved in most work, sport, and recreational activities; (3) uses the same exercise equipment for testing and training; (4) uses the same exercise technique for testing and training; (5) involves progressively increasing weightloads; (6) requires ten controlled repetitions (75% of maximum weightload); (7) can be completed in less than ten minutes; (8) can be expressed as a percentage of bodyweight; and (9) requires a single test administrator (Westcott 1988j).

The YMCA Leg Extension Test meets all of these criteria and is norm-referenced on over 900 men and women (Westcott 1986i). The evaluation procedures and scoring system are presented in Appendix F. Although strength development is specific to individual muscle groups, the quadriceps are reasonably representative of one's strength fitness. Consequently, improved test scores motivate most members to continue their training efforts.

Self-Recording

Self-recording is a simple but successful means for motivating members. Regular record keeping tends to promote program adherence, whether dieting, running, or strength training. Perhaps this is because a self-recording card reminds the exerciser of previous training efforts, making it psychologically more difficult to miss a workout. Also, the self-recording card indicates past improvement, which serves as an incentive for continued training. It is therefore advisable to have members maintain an accurate exercise record, and to check their self-recording card periodically. Appendix E presents a sample strength training logbook.

Supervised Training

One of the best means for motivating members is supervised training sessions. If we have learned anything about training effectiveness, we know that individuals work more conscientiously when someone is overseeing the exercise session. That is, they exhibit better training technique and greater exercise effort, both of which enhance strength development. Because training results and training motivation are closely related, members should be encouraged to take supervised exercise sessions on a regular basis.

In addition to better results, supervised training provides more opportunities for instructor feedback and reinforcement. Positive and productive interaction between instructors and members is an important motivating factor. Generally speaking, members who participate in supervised training sessions seem less likely to discontinue their exercise program.

Role Modeling

Strength training instructors are automatically models of behavior for their program participants, and especially for new members. Staff behavior sets a powerful example for members in many respects. First, instructors should always demonstrate proper form when using the equipment. The better technique they use, the better technique members tend to use.

Second, instructors should always exhibit a positive attitude when they are on duty. When staff show that they enjoy their work, members are more likely to enjoy their workouts.

Third, instructors should always conduct themselves in a professional manner. When staff are friendly, courteous, and respectful, members tend to treat each other the same way.

One goal of good instructors is to change sedentary adults into exercising adults. According to a questionnaire survey distributed throughout New England (Westcott 1986m), fitness participants desire three key qualities in their instructors. In order of priority these are: (1) knowledge in exercise science, (2) teaching skills, and (3) enthusiasm. That is, new exercisers want to work with instructors who understand physical fitness and who can communicate exercise concepts in a relevant and enthusiastic manner.

Staff Selection

It would be difficult to overstate the importance of high-quality instructors. However, many strength training facilities have difficulty hiring competent and caring staff members. It is not easy to find full-time instructors who have high levels of knowledge, teaching skills and enthusiasm, and it is even harder to locate part-time instructors with these qualities.

So where does one start? One approach is to hire the most qualified applicants in terms of education and experience. Although knowledge of exercise science may be the most important instructor characteristic, it is probably the most easily acquired. That is, most reasonably intelligent people can learn the principles and practices of sensible strength training. However, it appears considerably more difficult to develop effective teaching skills and genuine enthusiasm toward participants.

Consequently, one criterion for staff selection is a sincere desire to help people become physically fit. Good instructors are just as enthusiastic about their members' exercise efforts as they are about their own fitness achievements. Good instructors like to interact with participants, give teaching suggestions, and reinforce personal progress. They also like to learn more about fitness and seek opportunities to increase their fitness knowledge.

One excellent source for new full-time staff is a student internship program. Those interns whose fitness philosophy is consistent with the organization and who display desirable instructor characteristics usually make an easy transition to professional staff responsibilities.

Staff Training

Once potential staff members have been identified, it is essential to give them specialized training. Regardless of background and abilities it is best to assume that every applicant can benefit from a structured staff training program. The staff training program should help each new instructor learn more about fitness, develop better teaching skills, and become more encouraging toward participants.

Because full-time fitness directors typically have diverse job descriptions with numerous responsibilities, this section addresses staff training for part-time strength instructors.

At one strength fitness facility each new instructor is scheduled for a two-hour introductory session. During this meeting, the strength training director presents the following information and materials:

Step 1:   Necessary paperwork for payroll and administrative purposes.

Step 2:   Personal copy of strength training textbook which serves as the major information resource.

Step 3:   Relevant strength training articles, especially pertaining to exercise principles, training procedures, and instructional technique.

Step 4:   Instructor manual containing sections on job description, general staff expectations, specific instructor responsibilities, new member orientation, emergency procedures, and employment agreement.

Step 5:   Slide presentation on strength training benefits, strength training research, strength training principles, and strength training procedures.

Additional two-hour training sessions are scheduled for hands-on exercise instruction. During these sessions the strength training director puts the new instructor on each exercise machine and explains proper training technique. The roles are then reversed, and the new instructor teaches each exercise machine to the strength training director. By so doing, the new instructor develops both teaching skills and confidence prior to working with members.

The next step is to schedule the new instructor on several shifts with senior staff. This allows the new instructor to function independently but have the security of an experienced staff member in case any assistance is needed.

If all goes well to this point, the new instructor is allowed to take full responsibility for the members training under his/her direction. Monthly staff meetings and regular training updates provide ongoing learning opportunities for all strength fitness instructors.

Staff Behavior

Appropriate staff behavior may vary from facility to facility. For example, some facilities may require staff to wear special uniforms while others may prefer instructors to wear business clothes when working with members. Given a certain degree of individualism among staff members, consider seven basic guidelines for on-duty behavior.

Be a Role Model

Staff members should make a conscious effort to model both the exercise and social behaviors they expect from their members. That is, they should follow facility guidelines, use proper exercise form, strive for a high level of personal fitness, and treat all members with courtesy and respect.

No Food, Drink, or Papers

It is important for all instructors to have occasional breaks to relax, have a snack, or otherwise recharge their batteries. However, it is not desirable for staff to be eating a sandwich, drinking a soda, or reading a newspaper when they should be actively supervising the strength training facility.

No Statues, No Flirts

There are basically two extremes among instructors. At one end are those who just stand around as if they were statues, never speaking unless spoken to first. At the other end are those who spend inordinate amounts of time with particular members, carrying on endless and often unwanted conversations. Neither type of staff is helpful to the general membership or beneficial to the facility management.

Make Contact With Members

Perhaps the most important responsibility of an instructor is to make contact with members. In fact, this is the main reason for having a supervised fitness facility. Most members appreciate a few minutes of instructor interaction. Questions, answers, feedback, and reinforcement are just a few reasons most exercise participants prefer training in facilities that have competent and personable instructors.

Check Form and Progress

One of the most productive uses of an instructor's time is to check members' exercise form and fitness progress. Observing participants as they train and reviewing their workout cards generally helps them to attain better results. Because most members are interested in personal achievement, this type of instructor interaction is both meaningful and motivational.

Act Positive and Professional

It is important that staff conduct themselves in a positive and professional manner regardless of circumstances. Every member, cooperative or difficult, timid or bold, should be treated with courtesy and respect. Performance feedback should be given in an encouraging tone, and inappropriate behavior should be dealt with professionally rather than emotionally. It is important that the strength training facility be characterized by a positive and pleasant atmosphere. This is only possible when the instructors are positive and professional toward members and toward each other.

Keep the Strength Training Facility Clean

Members appreciate a clean facility and smooth running equipment. Although daily maintenance and cleaning is usually scheduled during off-use or low-use hours, it is most necessary during high-use periods. Consequently, every instructor should be alert to facility cleanliness and equipment function. Dust, dirt, squeaks, and misplaced items should be dealt with the minute they are observed, even if an instructor must excuse herself for a moment. Keeping the facility clean and the equipment polished is one of the most visible ways to demonstrate a caring attitude toward members.

Activity Programming

While most well-managed facilities have plenty of participants before work, during the lunch hour, and after work, few are busy throughout the day. The low-use periods provide excellent opportunities to work with specialized groups. This type of homogeneous grouping is helpful to the individuals involved, especially those who would otherwise feel self-conscious in the strength training facility. Activity programming is also a way to make better use of the facility, equipment, and instructional staff.

There are basically three low-use periods during typical weekdays. These are mid-morning (approximately 9 A.M. to 11 A.M.), midafternoon (approximately 1 P.M. to 4 P.M.), and late evening (approximately 7 P.M. to 9 P.M.). At one strength fitness facility, these low-use periods are programmed with the following group activities (see table 6.3).

Cardiac Rehabilitation Program

The cardiac rehabilitation program is a medically supervised class that exercises from 8 A.M. to 9 A.M. Monday, Wednesday, and Friday in the indoor track area. At the completion of class, the cardiologist sends selected members to the strength training facility. Working closely with the strength training staff, these participants perform conservative muscular conditioning between 9 A.M. and 10 A.M. on the strength training equipment.

Morning Weight Loss Program

One of the most popular group activities is a weight loss program that includes a heart healthy diet, weekly nutrition lectures, endurance training, and strength training. The morning class exercises Monday, Wednesday, and Friday from 10 A.M. to 11 A.M. in the strength training facility.

Senior Fitness Program

This program is limited to men and women over sixty years of age. The participants perform about twenty minutes of strength exercise and about twenty minutes of endurance exercise on a Tuesday, Thursday, Saturday sequence. The 10 A.M. to 11 A.M. time frame seems to work well for those seniors who are not employed.

Physical Rehabilitation Program

Although the strength fitness facility houses a professionally staffed physical therapy center, it also provides a physical rehabilitation program during the early afternoon. This program is conducted by a certified staff member and is designed for persons who have completed physical therapy but are not yet able to exercise on their own. Participants include victims of strokes, automobile accidents, athletic injuries, and various disabling diseases.

Sports Fitness Program

The strength training facility is home to many high school athletic teams for off-season conditioning programs. Depending on the season, cross-country, basketball, football, track, and swim teams perform circuit strength training between 3 P.M. and 4 P.M. on a Monday, Wednesday, Friday schedule. Although the program is conducted by the instructional staff, the head coach is usually present for motivational purposes.

Youth Fitness Program

Geared more for nonathletes, the youth fitness program provides carefully supervised strength training for boys and girls between nine and fourteen years of age. Like the sports fitness program, it is scheduled from 3 P.M. to 4 P.M., but on Tuesdays, Thursdays, and Saturdays. In an attempt to form healthy lifestyles, the youth fitness program includes strength training, endurance training, and weekly slide presentations on exercise and nutrition.

Evening Weight Loss Program

This program is identical to the morning weight loss program except for the exercise time, which is Monday, Wednesday, and Friday from 7 P.M. to 8 P.M.

Ski-Golf-Tennis Preparation Program

The intent of this program is to prepare skiers (fall and winter) and golf-tennis players (spring and summer) for safe and successful activity participation. It is designed for comprehensive muscle conditioning to reduce the risk of injuries and to enhance performance power. The ski-golf-tennis program is conducted from 7 P.M. to 8 P.M. on a Tuesday, Thursday, Saturday schedule.

Table 6.3   Group activities scheduled for facility low-use periods.

Mornings		
9 A.M. – 10 A.M.	MWF	Cardiac rehabilitation program
10 A.M. – 11 A.M.	MWF	Morning weight loss program
10 A.M. – 11 A.M.	TThS	Senior fitness program
Afternoons		
1 P.M. – 3 P.M.	MWF	Physical rehabilitation program
3 P.M. – 4 P.M.	MWF	Sports fitness program
3 P.M. – 4 P.M.	TThS	Youth fitness program
Evenings		
7 P.M. – 8 P.M.	MWF	Evening weight loss program
7 P.M. – 8 P.M.	TThS	Ski-golf-tennis preparation program

Seven

Strength Training Exercises

Strength training exercises should be selected on the basis of safety and effectiveness. In terms of safety, each exercise should have a low risk of injury when performed properly. In terms of effectiveness, each exercise should permit a progressive strength stimulus to the target muscle groups.

The forty-three exercises illustrated in this chapter meet these criteria. The first section describes a representative exercise for each of the major muscle groups using single station weightstack machines. The second section presents similar exercises performed on single station pneumatic (compressed air) machines. The third section highlights some basic exercises utilizing free-weight (barbell and dumbbell) equipment. The fourth section discusses exercises common to multi-station weightstack machines. The fifth section addresses three key exercises performed with body resistance, and the last section examines some specialized exercises for the legs and forearms.

When muscles act upon a single joint, the resulting movement is curvilinear (curved). Consequently, exercises that involve a single joint action produce rotary movements and are referred to as rotary exercises. When muscles act upon two or more joints, the resulting movement is typically linear (straight), even though the individual joint movements are curvilinear. Consequently, exercises that involve two or more joint actions generally produce linear movements and are referred to as linear exercises.

The exercises are presented from larger muscle groups to smaller muscle groups, and should be performed in this order whenever possible. Each exercise should be executed with strict technique through a full range of joint movement.

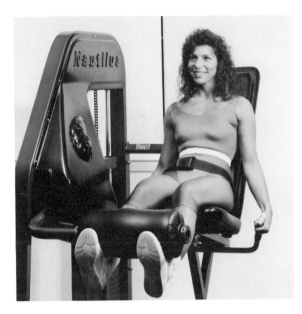

Figure 7.1 Leg extension

Exercises Performed on Single Station Weightstack Machines

Leg Extension Machine

As illustrated in figure 7.1, the leg extension is a rotary exercise that largely isolates the quadriceps muscles. The quadriceps muscles are responsible for extending the knee and assist in flexing the hip.

Technical Points:

1. Sit on seat and align knee joint with machine axis of rotation.
2. Use additional pad for back support if necessary.
3. Fasten seat belt.
4. Place hands on handgrips.
5. Place ankles in neutral position behind lever arm.
6. Slowly lift lever arm until the quadriceps are fully contracted and hold momentarily.
7. Slowly lower lever arm until plates almost touch weightstack, and repeat.

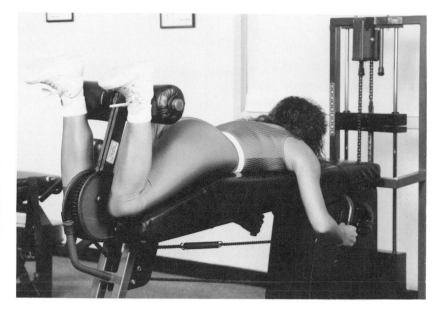

Figure 7.2 Leg curl

Note: By not allowing the plates to rest on the weightstack, muscle tension is maintained throughout the exercise set.

Leg Curl Machine

As shown in figure 7.2, the leg curl is a rotary exercise that largely isolates the hamstring muscles. The hamstring muscles are responsible for flexing the knee and assist in extending the hip.

Technical Points:

1. Lie on seat and align knee joint with machine axis of rotation.
2. Place hands on handgrips.
3. Place ankles in neutral position behind lever arm.
4. Slowly lift lever arm until the hamstrings are fully contracted and hold momentarily.
5. Slowly lower lever arm until plates almost touch weightstack and repeat.

Note: For complete contraction of the hamstring muscles, the hips must raise slightly off the support pad, but should be supported as much as possible.

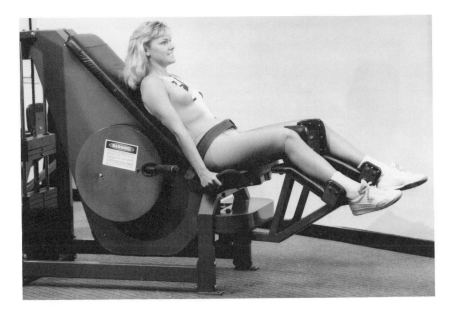

Figure 7.3 Hip adduction

Hip Adduction Machine

As shown in figure 7.3, the hip adduction is a rotary exercise in which the hip joint is the axis of rotation. The hip adductor muscles adduct the legs toward the midline of the body.

Technical Points:

1. Sit on seat with back fully supported.
2. Fasten seat belt.
3. Place hands on handgrips.
4. Place legs outside knee and ankle pads.
5. Slowly move legs together and hold momentarily in final position.
6. Slowly move legs apart until comfortably stretched and repeat.

Note: Assistance may be necessary to place the legs into the starting position.

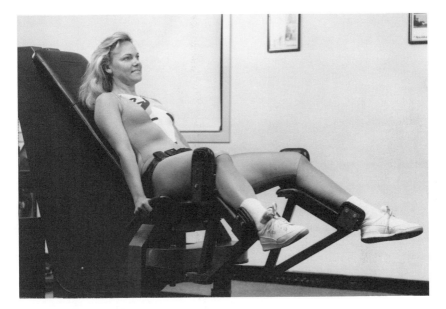

Figure 7.4 Hip abduction

Hip Abduction Machine

As presented in figure 7.4, the hip abduction is a rotary exercise in which the hip joint is the axis of rotation. The hip abductor muscles abduct the legs away from the midline of the body.

Technical Points:

1. Sit on seat.
2. Fasten seat belt.
3. Place hands on handgrips.
4. Place legs inside knee and ankle pads.
5. Slowly move legs apart and hold momentarily in final position.
6. Slowly move legs together until plates almost touch weightstack, and repeat.

Note: It is important to attain a full range of movement in this exercise.

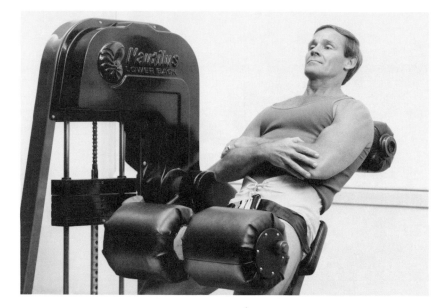

Figure 7.5 Back extension

Low Back Machine

As illustrated in figure 7.5, the back extension is a rotary exercise that emphasizes the low back muscles. The low back muscles are responsible for trunk extension.

Technical Points:

1.   Sit on seat in front of lever arm with feet evenly spaced on floor grid.
2.   Fasten seat belt and secure thigh pads.
3.   Fold arms across chest and keep head in neutral position.
4.   Slowly push lever arm backward to extended position and pause momentarily.
5.   Return slowly until plates almost touch weightstack, and repeat.

Note: It is important to perform all lower back movements slowly.

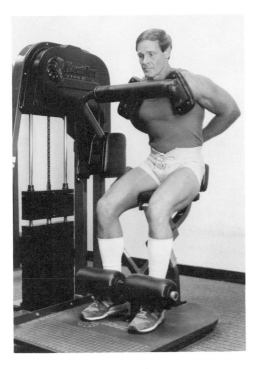

Figure 7.6 Abdominal curl

Abdominal Machine

As shown in figure 7.6, the abdominal curl is a rotary exercise that emphasizes the abdominal muscles. The abdominal muscles are responsible for trunk flexion.

Technical Points:

1. Sit on seat behind torso pads, with feet secured beneath foot rollers.
2. Place hands behind back.
3. Slowly push lever arm forward about thirty degrees, and pause momentarily.
4. Return slowly until plates almost touch weightstack, and repeat.

Note: The seat should be adjusted so that the top of the torso pads are a little higher than the shoulders.

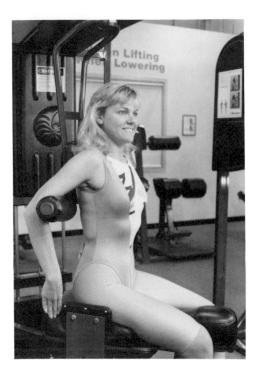

Figure 7.7 Rotary torso

Rotary Torso Machine

As illustrated in figure 7.7, the rotary torso is a rotary exercise that addresses the oblique muscles. These muscles enable rotational movements in the midsection area.

Technical Points:

1. Sit on seat with back straight and in line with machine axis of rotation.
2. Place arms behind roller pads.
3. With head, shoulders, and torso in a fixed position, turn slowly toward the right, about forty-five degrees past the neutral position.
4. After a momentary pause, slowly return to starting position.
5. Repeat this movement pattern until fatigued and slowly return plates to weightstack.

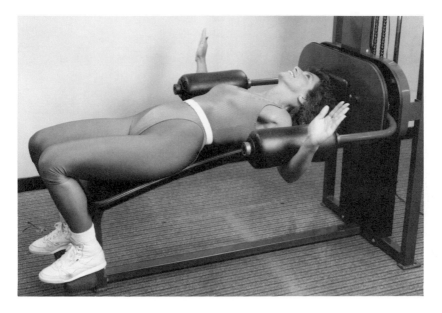

Figure 7.8 Ten-degree chest

6.   Change seat position and repeat the above procedures moving toward the left.

Note: It is important to maintain a vertical back position throughout this exercise.

Ten-Degree Chest Machine

As presented in figure 7.8, the ten-degree chest is a rotary exercise that emphasizes the pectoralis major and anterior deltoid muscles. These muscles are prime movers for horizontal shoulder flexion.

Technical Points:

1.   Lie on seat with feet on floor, foot rest, or stool.
2.   Place upper arms under roller pads.
3.   Slowly raise roller pads until they meet directly above chest and hold momentarily.
4.   Slowly lower roller pads until plates almost touch weight-stack, and repeat.

Note: The head, shoulders, and hips should remain on the seat throughout the exercise.

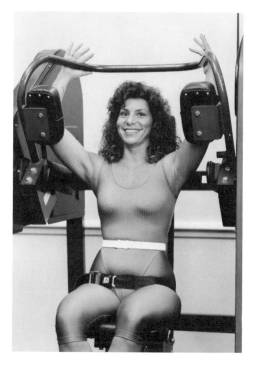

Figure 7.9 Pullover

Pullover Machine

As illustrated in figure 7.9, the pullover is a rotary exercise that emphasizes the latissimus dorsi, upper back, and posterior deltoid muscles. These muscles are prime movers for shoulder extension.

Technical Points:

1. Sit on seat and align shoulder joints with machine axis of rotation.
2. Reposition seat or use additional pad as necessary.
3. Fasten seat belt.
4. Press foot lever to bring arm pads into position.
5. Place upper arms against arm pads, and grip movement bar lightly with hands.
6. Slowly bring movement bar downward until it contacts seat belt and pause momentarily.
7. Slowly bring movement bar upward until muscles are comfortably stretched, and repeat.

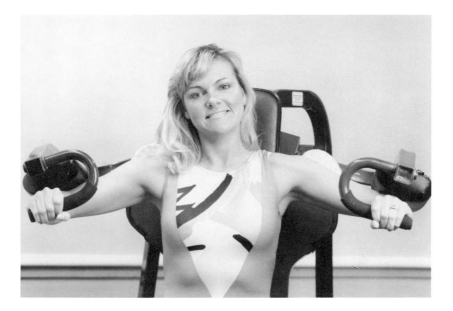

Figure 7.10 Lateral raise

8. After final repetition, press foot lever to disengage arms and lower plates to weightstack.

Note: The downward movement should be acccompanied by a slight trunk flexion to maintain support behind the lower back. The major movement force should come from the upper arms rather than from the hands.

Lateral Raise Machine

As presented in figure 7.10, the lateral raise is a rotary exercise that largely isolates the deltoid (anterior, middle, and posterior) muscles. The deltoid muscles are prime movers for shoulder abduction.

Technical Points:

1. Sit on seat and align shoulder joints with machine axes of rotation.
2. Reposition seat or use additional pad as necessary.
3. Fasten seat belt.

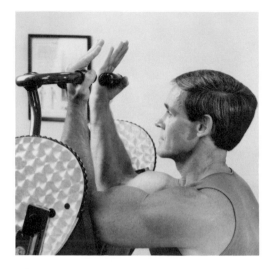

Figure 7.11 Biceps curl

4. Place upper arms against arm pads and grip handles loosely.
5. Slowly lift arm pads to shoulder level and hold momentarily.
6. Slowly lower arm pads until arms almost touch sides, and repeat.

Note: Keep the back straight and the head in neutral position throughout the exercise. By not letting the arms rest on the sides, constant tension is maintained on the shoulder muscles.

Biceps Curl Machine

As presented in figure 7.11, the biceps curl is a rotary exercise that largely isolates the biceps muscles. The biceps muscles flex the elbows and supinate the wrists.

Technical Points:

1. Sit on seat and place elbows on pad in line with machine axes of rotation.
2. Reposition seat or use additional pad as necessary.
3. Hold handles with loose, underhand grip.

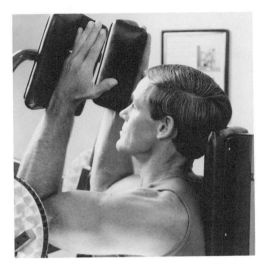

Figure 7.12 Triceps extension

4. Slowly lift handles until elbows are fully flexed and hold momentarily.
5. Slowly lower handles until elbows are nearly extended, and repeat.

Note: The shoulders should be positioned level with the elbows.

Triceps Extension Machine

As shown in figure 7.12, the triceps extension is a rotary exercise that largely isolates the triceps muscles. The triceps muscles extend the elbows.

Technical Points:

1. Sit on seat and place the elbows on pad in line with machine axes of rotation.
2. Reposition seat or use additional pad as necessary.
3. Place side of hands on hand pads.
4. Slowly press hand pads forward until elbows are fully extended and hold momentarily.
5. Slowly return hand pads until elbows are comfortably flexed, and repeat.

Note: The shoulders should be positioned level with the elbows. It is important to keep the elbows on the pad at all times during the exercise.

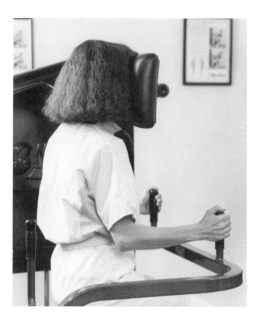

Figure 7.13 Neck flexion

Neck Flexion Machine

As presented in figure 7.13, the neck flexion is a rotary exercise about the cervical vertebrae. The neck flexor muscles are prime movers for neck flexion.

Technical Points:

1. Sit on seat and place face in center of head pads.
2. Reposition seat or use additional pad as necessary.
3. Place hands loosely on handgrips.
4. Slowly move head forward until neck is fully flexed and pause momentarily.
5. Slowly move head backward until neck is comfortably extended, and repeat.

Note: It is important to maintain the torso in an erect position throughout the exercise.

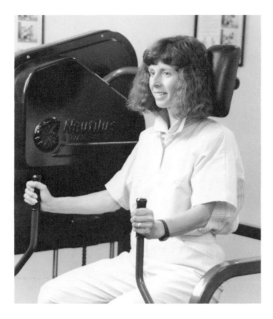

Figure 7.14 Neck extension

Neck Extension Machine

As presented in figure 7.14, the neck extension is a rotary exercise about the cervical vertebrae. The neck extensor muscles are prime movers for neck extension.

Technical Points:

1. Sit on seat and place head in center of head pads.
2. Reposition seat or use additional pad as necessary.
3. Place hands loosely on handgrips.
4. Slowly move head backward until neck is comfortably extended and hold momentarily.
5. Slowly move head forward until neck is comfortably flexed, and repeat.

Note: It is important to maintain the torso in an erect position throughout the exercise.

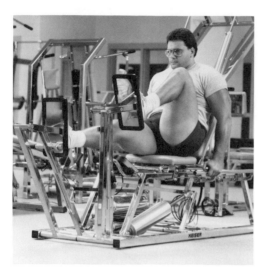

Figure 7.15 Leg press

Exercises Performed on Single Station Pneumatic Machines

Leg Press Machine

As illustrated in figure 7.15, the leg press is a linear exercise for the quadriceps, hamstrings, and gluteal muscles. These muscles work together to produce simultaneous knee extension and hip extension.

Technical Points:

1. Sit down and place feet in middle of foot pads with legs parallel to floor when fully extended.
2. Adjust sliding lock bar for unilateral (one leg) or bilateral (both legs) training.
3. Hold the handgrips and push footpads forward by extending the legs.
4. At the completion of the exercise engage the stop bar and allow the foot pads to rest against the roller stops.
5. Perform each repetition through a full range of joint movement in a controlled manner.

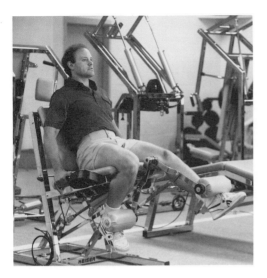

Figure 7.16 Leg extension

Notes: Keep the knees in line with the shoulders throughout the exercise. To increase resistance press the right thumb button and to decrease resistance press the left thumb button. Never increase resistance when the knees are in a locked position.

Leg Extension Machine

As illustrated in figure 7.16, the leg extension is a rotary exercise that largely isolates the quadriceps muscles. The quadriceps muscles are responsible for extending the knee and assist in flexing the hip.

Technical Points:

1. Sit down and adjust seat so that the knees are in line with the machine axis of rotation.
2. Place ankles behind the roller pads.
3. Grasp the handgrips and extend the knees either unilaterally or bilaterally.
4. Perform each repetition through a full range of joint movement in a controlled manner.

Note: To increase resistance press the right thumb button and to decrease resistance press the left thumb button.

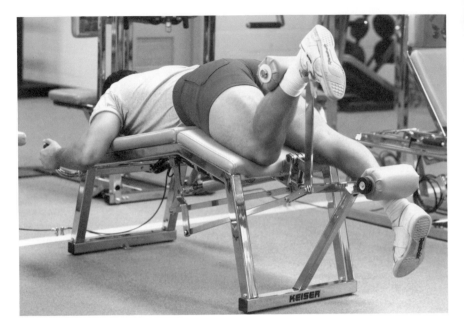

Figure 7.17 Leg curl

Leg Curl Machine

As shown in figure 7.17, the leg curl is a rotary exercise that largely isolates the hamstrings muscles. The hamstring muscles are responsible for flexing the knee and assist in extending the hip.

Technical Points:

1. Lie flat on pad with knees in line with machine axis of rotation.
2. Place ankles under the roller pads.
3. Grasp the handgrips and flex the knees either unilaterally or bilaterally.
4. Perform each repetition through a full range of joint movement in a controlled manner.

Note: To increase resistance press the right thumb button and to decrease resistance press the left thumb button.

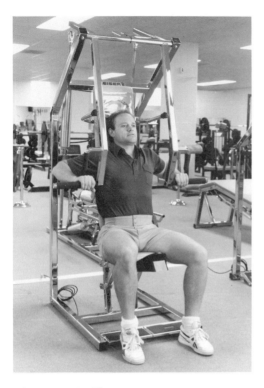

Figure 7.18 Chest press

Chest Press Machine

As shown in figure 7.18, the chest press is a linear exercise that involves the pectoralis major, anterior deltoid, and triceps muscles. The pectoralis major and anterior deltoid muscles are prime movers for horizontal shoulder flexion. The triceps muscles are prime movers for elbow extension.

Technical Points:
1. Sit down and adjust seat so that the handgrips are at chest level.
2. Select one of the two handgrips and push lever arms forward either unilaterally or bilaterally.
3. Perform each repetition through a full range of joint movement in a controlled manner.

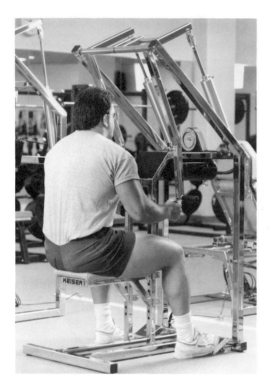

Figure 7.19 Upper back machine

Notes: To increase resistance press the right foot pedal and to decrease resistance press the left foot pedal. Never increase resistance when the elbows are in a locked position.

Upper Back Machine

As illustrated in figure 7.19, the upper back machine provides a linear exercise for the latissimus dorsi, upper back, posterior deltoid, and biceps muscles. The latissimus dorsi, upper back, and posterior deltoid muscles are prime movers for shoulder extension. The biceps muscles are prime movers for elbow flexion.

Technical Points:

1. Sit down and adjust seat so that the handgrips are at shoulder level.
2. Select one of the two handgrips and pull lever arms backward either unilaterally or bilaterally.

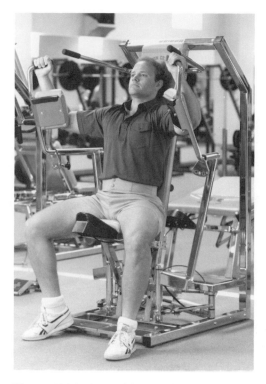

Figure 7.20 Seated butterfly

3. Perform each repetition through a full range of joint movement in a controlled manner.

Note: To increase resistance press the right foot pedal and to decrease resistance press the left foot pedal.

Seated Butterfly Machine

As shown in figure 7.20, the seated butterfly is a rotary exercise that emphasizes the pectoralis major and anterior deltoid muscles. These muscles are prime movers for horizontal shoulder flexion.

Technical Points:

1. Sit down and adjust seat so that the arms are parallel to the floor with forearms at right angles.
2. Place hands on handgrips and forearms against the movement pads.

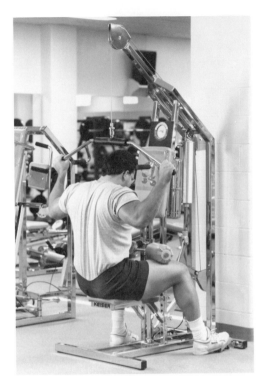

Figure 7.21 High lat pulldown

3. Squeeze the movement pads together across the chest.
4. Perform each repetition through a full range of joint movement in a controlled manner.

Notes: Keep the back firmly pressed against the seatback throughout the exercise. To increase resistance press the right foot pedal and to decrease resistance press the left foot pedal. Unilateral training is made possible by holding the overhead support bar with one arm while exercising the other arm.

High Lat Pulldown Machine

As illustrated in figure 7.21, the high lat pulldown is a linear exercise designed to work the latissimus dorsi, upper back, posterior deltoid, and biceps muscles. The latissimus dorsi, upper back, and posterior deltoid muscles are prime movers for shoulder extension. The biceps muscles are prime movers for elbow flexion.

Technical Points:

1. Sit down and adjust seat so that the arms are fully extended when holding the handgrips.
2. Secure thighs comfortably beneath the roller pads.
3. Grasp one of the two handgrips and pull bar down to shoulder level either in front or behind the head.
4. Perform each repetition through a full range of joint movement in a controlled manner.

Note: To increase resistance press the right foot pedal and to decrease resistance press the left foot pedal.

Military Press Machine

As shown in figure 7.22, the military press is a linear exercise that involves the deltoid (anterior, middle, and posterior), upper trapezius, and triceps muscles. The deltoid muscles are prime movers for shoulder abduction. The upper trapezius muscles are prime movers for shoulder elevation, and the triceps muscles are prime movers for elbow extension.

Technical Points:

1. Sit down and adjust seat so that the handgrips are slightly below the shoulders.
2. Grasp the handgrips and push lever arms upward either unilaterally or bilaterally.
3. Perform each repetition through a full range of joint movement in a controlled manner.

Notes: Keep the back firmly pressed against the seatback throughout the exercise. Do not allow the handgrips to contact the shoulders. To increase resistance press the right foot pedal and to decrease resistance press the left foot pedal. Never increase resistance when the elbows are in a locked position.

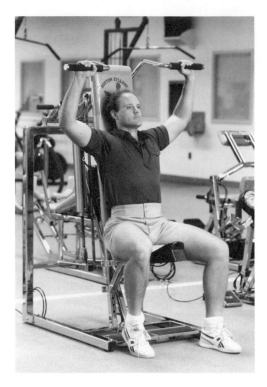

Figure 7.22 Military press

Arm Curl Machine

As shown in figure 7.23, the arm curl is a rotary exercise that emphasizes the biceps muscles. The biceps muscles flex the elbows and supinate the wrists.

Technical Points:

1. Sit down and adjust seat so that the elbows are in line with the machine axis of rotation.
2. Grasp handgrips loosely and flex the elbows either unilaterally or bilaterally.
3. Perform each repetition through a full range of joint movement in a controlled manner.

Notes: Keep the elbows in contact with the pads throughout the exercise. To increase resistance press the right foot pedal and to decrease resistance press the left foot pedal.

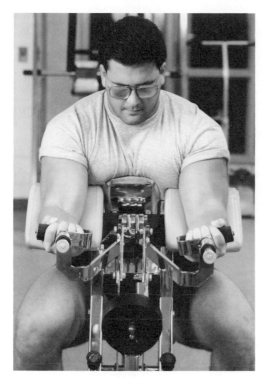

Figure 7.23 Arm curl

Tricep Machine

As illustrated in figure 7.24, the tricep machine provides a linear exercise for the triceps, pectoralis major, latissimus dorsi, and anterior deltoid muscles. The triceps muscles are prime movers for elbow extension. The pectoralis major and latissimus dorsi are prime movers for shoulder adduction, and the anterior deltoids are prime movers for shoulder flexion.

Technical Points:

1. Sit down and adjust seat so that the handgrips are at chest level.
2. Fasten seatbelt securely.
3. Grasp handgrips and press levers downward either unilaterally or bilaterally.
4. Perform each repetition through a full range of joint movement in a controlled manner.

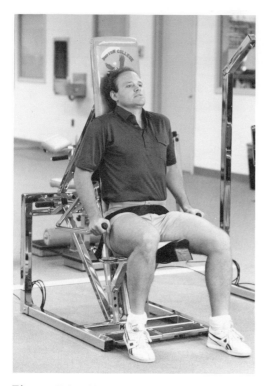

Figure 7.24 Tricep machine

Notes: Keep the back firmly pressed against the seatback throughout the exercise. To increase resistance press the right foot pedal and to decrease resistance press the left foot pedal. Never increase resistance when the elbows are in a locked position.

Exercises Performed with Free Weight Equipment

Squat

As illustrated in figure 7.25, the squat is a linear exercise that involves the quadriceps, hamstrings, and gluteal muscles. These muscles work together to produce simultaneous knee extension and hip extension.

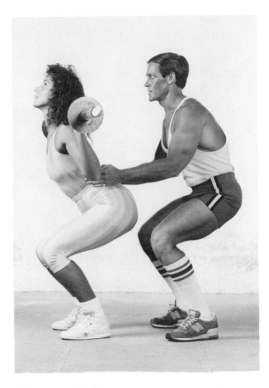

Figure 7.25 Squat

Technical Points:

1. Place barbell across the upper back, and lift it off the supporting rack.
2. Hands should be wide spaced, and feet should be shoulder width apart.
3. Slowly lower the body until the thighs are approximately parallel to the floor.
4. Slowly raise the body to a standing position, and repeat.
5. Keep the head up and the back straight throughout the exercise.

Note: It is important to incorporate a spotter or a safety rack when performing barbell squats.

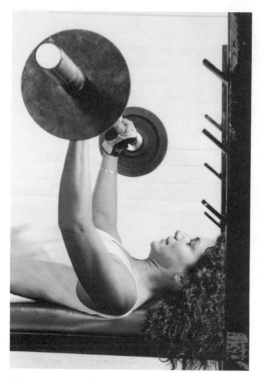

Figure 7.26 Bench press

Bench Press

As shown in figure 7.26, the bench press is a linear exercise that involves the pectoralis major, anterior deltoid, and triceps muscles. The pectoralis major and anterior deltoid muscles are prime movers for horizontal shoulder flexion. The triceps muscles are prime movers for elbow extension.

Technical Points:

1. Lie on bench with feet on floor.
2. Grasp barbell with hands slightly more than shoulder width apart.
3. Lift barbell from standards and hold in lockout position above chest.
4. Slowly lower barbell to chest.
5. Slowly press barbell up to lockout position, and repeat.

Note: The head, shoulders, and hips should remain on the bench throughout the exercise.

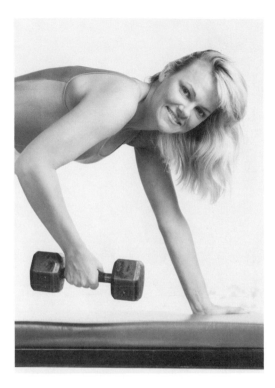

Figure 7.27 Bent row

Bent Row

As shown in figure 7.27, the bent row is a linear exercise that involves the latissimus dorsi, upper back, posterior deltoid, and biceps muscles. The latissimus dorsi, upper back, and posterior deltoid muscles are prime movers for shoulder extension. The biceps muscles are prime movers for elbow flexion.

Technical Points:

1. Bend at waist and place one hand on bench.
2. Grip dumbbell with other hand at full arm extension.
3. Slowly lift dumbbell to shoulder and hold momentarily.
4. Slowly lower dumbbell to full arm extension, and repeat.

Note: It is important to place one hand on a bench to support the upper body and reduce stress on the lower back.

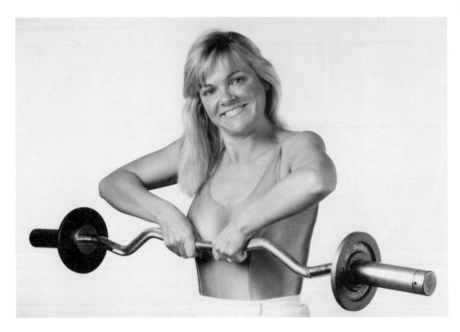

Figure 7.28 Upright row

Upright Row

As presented in figure 7.28, the upright row is a linear exercise that emphasizes the deltoid (anterior, middle, and posterior) and upper trapezius muscles. The deltoid muscles are prime movers for shoulder abduction. The upper trapezius muscles are prime movers for shoulder elevation.

Technical Points:
1. Hold bar with a close, overhand grip.
2. Slowly lift bar to chin with elbows leading and hold momentarily.
3. Slowly lower bar to full arm extension, and repeat.

Note: Head and torso should remain erect throughout this exercise.

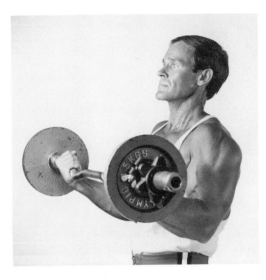

Figure 7.29 Biceps curl

Biceps Curl

As illustrated in figure 7.29, the biceps curl is a rotary exercise that emphasizes the biceps muscles. The biceps muscles flex the elbows and supinate the wrists.

Technical Points:

1. Hold barbell at full arm extension with a shoulder width, underhand grip.
2. Slowly curl bar to chest level and hold momentarily.
3. Slowly lower bar to starting position, and repeat.

Note: It is important to keep the torso erect and the elbows stabilized against the sides throughout the exercise.

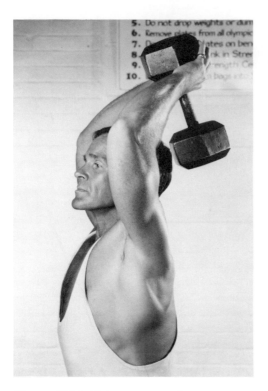

Figure 7.30 Triceps extension

Triceps Extension

As shown in figure 7.30, the triceps extension is a rotary exercise that emphasizes the triceps muscles. The triceps muscles extend the elbows.

Technical Points:

1. Hold dumbbell in both hands with arms extended overhead.
2. Keeping the elbows high, slowly lower dumbbell behind the neck.
3. Slowly lift dumbbell to starting position, and repeat.

Note: It is important to maintain good posture and to keep the elbows high throughout this exercise.

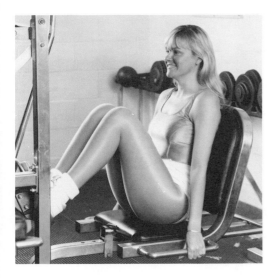

Figure 7.31 Leg press

Exercises Performed on Multi-Station Weightstack Machines

Leg Press Station

As illustrated in figure 7.31, the leg press is a linear exercise that involves the quadriceps, hamstrings, and gluteal muscles. These muscles work together to produce simultaneous knee extension and hip extension.

Technical Points:

1. Sit securely in seat with feet evenly placed on foot pads.
2. Slowly push foot pads forward by extending the legs.
3. Slowly return to starting position, and repeat.

Note: The hips and low back should remain firmly pressed against the seat throughout the exercise.

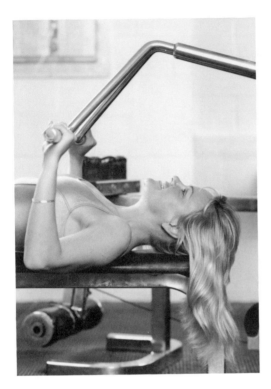

Figure 7.32 Bench press

Bench Press Station

As shown in figure 7.32, the bench press is a linear exercise that works the pectoralis major, anterior deltoid, and triceps muscles. The pectoralis major and anterior deltoid muscles are prime movers for horizontal shoulder flexion. The triceps muscles are prime movers for elbow extension.

Technical Points:

1. Lie on bench with feet on floor and hands comfortably spaced on handles.
2. Slowly push handles upward by extending the arms, and pause momentarily in lockout position.
3. Slowly lower handles to starting position, and repeat.

Note: The head, shoulders, and hips should remain on the bench throughout the exercise.

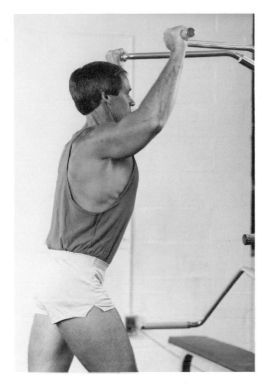

Figure 7.33 Overhead press

Overhead Press Station

As illustrated in figure 7.33, the overhead press is a linear exercise that involves the deltoid (anterior, middle, and posterior), upper trapezius, and triceps muscles. The deltoid muscles are prime movers for shoulder abduction. The upper trapezius muscles are prime movers for shoulder elevation, and the triceps muscles are prime movers for elbow extension.

Technical Points:

1. Assume staggered stance with hands comfortably spaced on handles.
2. Slowly push handles upward by extending the arms, and pause momentarily in the lockout position.
3. Slowly lower handles to starting position, and repeat.

Note: The back should remain as straight as possible throughout the exercise.

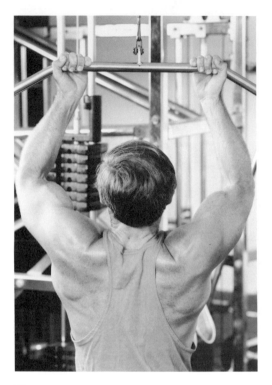

Figure 7.34 Lat pulldown

Lat Pulldown Station

As illustrated in figure 7.34, the lat pulldown is a linear exercise that works the latissimus dorsi, upper back, posterior deltoid, and biceps muscles. The latissimus dorsi, upper back, and posterior deltoid muscles are prime movers for shoulder extension. The biceps muscles are prime movers for elbow flexion.

Technical Points:

1. Kneel on floor and hold bar with an underhand grip.
2. Slowly pull bar to chest and pause momentarily.
3. Slowly return bar to starting position, and repeat.

Note: The back should remain as straight as possible throughout the exercise.

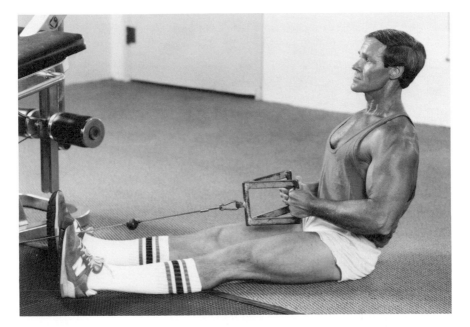

Figure 7.35 Low row

Low Row Station

As shown in figure 7.35, the low row is a linear exercise that works the latissimus dorsi, upper back, posterior deltoid, and biceps muscles. The latissimus dorsi, upper back, and posterior deltoid muscles are prime movers for horizontal shoulder extension. The biceps muscles are prime movers for elbow flexion.

Technical Points:

1. Sit on floor and hold bar with an overhand grip.
2. Slowly pull bar to chest and pause momentarily.
3. Slowly return bar to starting position, and repeat.

Note: The back should remain vertical throughout the exercise.

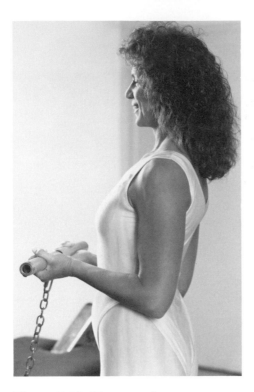

Figure 7.36 Biceps curl

Biceps Curl Station

As illustrated in figure 7.36, the biceps curl is a rotary exercise that emphasizes the biceps muscles. The biceps muscles flex the elbows and supinate the wrists.

Technical Points:

1. Assume shoulder width stance and hold bar with an underhand grip.
2. Slowly curl bar to chest level and pause momentarily.
3. Slowly lower bar to starting position, and repeat.

Note: It is important to keep the torso erect and the elbows stabilized against the sides throughout the exercise.

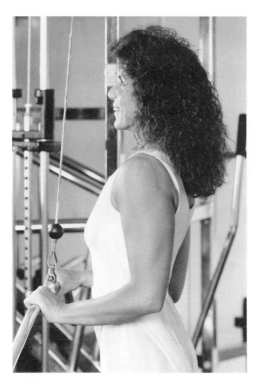

Figure 7.37 Triceps pressdown

Triceps Pressdown Station

As illustrated in figure 7.37, the triceps pressdown is a rotary exercise that emphasizes the triceps muscles. The triceps muscles extend the elbows.

Technical Points:

1. Assume shoulder width stance and hold bar with a close, overhand grip.
2. Bring bar to starting position below chin.
3. Slowly press bar downward until elbows are fully extended.
4. Slowly return bar to starting position, and repeat.

Note: It is important to keep the torso erect and the elbows stabilized against the sides throughout the exercise.

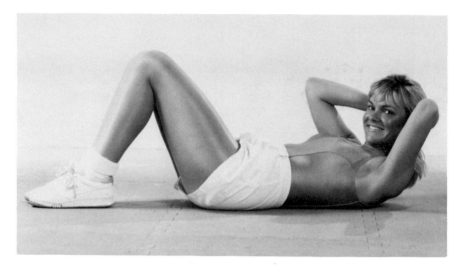

Figure 7.38 Trunk curl

Exercises Performed with Bodyweight Resistance

Trunk Curl

As illustrated in figure 7.38, the trunk curl is a rotary exercise that emphasizes the abdominal muscles. The abdominal muscles are responsible for trunk flexion.

Technical Points:

1. Lie on floor with knees bent and hands placed loosely on the head.
2. Slowly curl the head and shoulders forward and upward until the low back is pressed firmly against the floor.
3. Pause momentarily, return slowly to starting position, and repeat.

Notes: To produce more stress on the abdominal muscles and less stress on the lower back, be sure not to lift the low back off the floor as in a situp. Because the movement range is rather short, trunk curls should be performed very slowly.

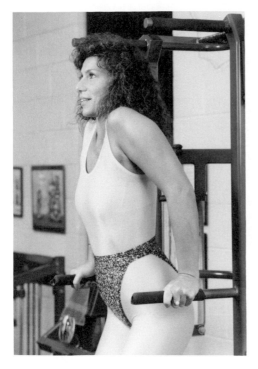

Figure 7.39 Bar dip

Bar Dip

As presented in figure 7.39, the bar dip is a linear exercise that involves the pectoralis major, latissimus dorsi, anterior deltoid, and triceps muscles. The pectoralis major and latissimus dorsi muscles are prime movers for shoulder adduction. The anterior deltoid muscles are prime movers for shoulder flexion, and the triceps muscles are prime movers for elbow extension.

Technical Points:
1. Begin exercise with arms fully extended in a lockout position.
2. Slowly lower body until upper arms are parallel to floor.
3. Slowly press body upward until arms are fully extended, and repeat.

Notes: This exercise should be performed with a straight body and a neutral head position. Resistance can be increased by attaching weights around the waist, thereby making the bar dip a free-weight exercise.

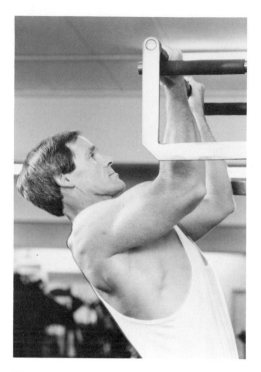

Figure 7.40 Pull-up

Pull-Up

As presented in figure 7.40, the pull-up is a linear exercise that involves the latissimus dorsi, upper back, posterior deltoid, and biceps muscles. The latissimus dorsi, upper back, and posterior deltoid muscles are prime movers for shoulder extension. The biceps muscles are prime movers for elbow flexion.

Technical Points:

1. Begin exercise with hands about shoulder width apart and elbows fully extended.
2. Slowly lift body until chin is well above bar and hold momentarily.
3. Slowly lower body to fully extended position, and repeat.

Notes: This exercise should be performed with a relatively straight body and a neutral head position. Resistance can be increased by attaching weights around the waist, thereby making the pull-up a free-weight exercise.

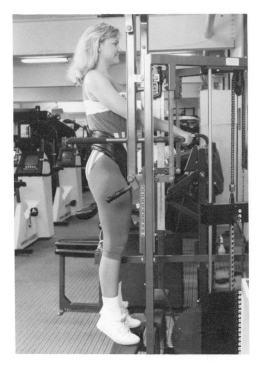

Figure 7.41 Heel raise

Exercises for the Legs and Forearms

Heel Raise

As illustrated in figure 7.41, the heel raise is a rotary exercise that emphasizes the calf muscles. The calf muscles extend the ankle joint.

Technical Points:
1. Stand with ball of foot on edge of step.
2. Place weightbelt over hips.
3. Hold handgrips loosely for balance.
4. Slowly lift body until ankles are fully extended and pause momentarily.
5. Slowly lower body until ankles are comfortably flexed, and repeat.

Note: Due to the short movement range, it is important to perform this exercise very slowly.

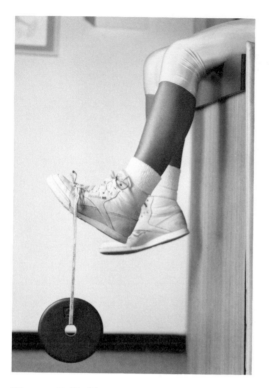

Figure 7.42 Toe raise

Toe Raise

As shown in figure 7.42, the toe raise is a rotary exercise that emphasizes the shin muscles. The shin muscles flex the ankle joint.

Technical Points:

1. Sit on high table with leg in vertical position.
2. Attach weight to toe area with shoestring.
3. Slowly lift toe toward shin until ankle is fully flexed and hold momentarily.
4. Slowly lower toe until ankle is comfortably extended, and repeat.

Note: Due to the short movement range, it is important to perform this exercise very slowly.

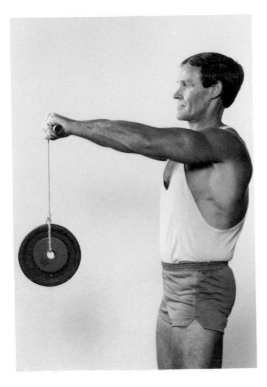

Figure 7.43 Wrist roll

Wrist Roll

As illustrated in figure 7.43, the wrist roll is a rotary exercise that emphasizes the forearm flexors during the lifting phase and the forearm extensors during the lowering phase. The forearm flexor muscles flex the wrist and the forearm extensor muscles extend the wrist.

Technical Points:

1. Hold roller bar in front of shoulders with overhand grip.
2. Slowly turn roller bar clockwise, alternating left hand and right hand until rope winds weight to top position.
3. Slowly turn roller bar counterclockwise, alternating left hand and right hand until rope unwinds weight to bottom position.

Note: Roller bar should be turned as far as possible with each hand. Rope should not be allowed to slip during the lowering phase.

Eight

Strength Training Concerns and Considerations

The preceding seven chapters of this text have presented essential information on strength training and muscle development. The first three chapters discussed the general benefits of strength fitness, basic muscle physiology, movement mechanics, and strength performance factors. Chapter 4 addressed relevant research in the areas of training variables and training responses. Chapter 5 incorporated the research findings into the principles and recommendations for sensible strength training.

Because application of knowledge is the most critical aspect of strength training, considerable attention was given to program design and facility management in chapter 6. Finally, a chapter on strength exercises explained and illustrated safe and effective training procedures for a variety of strength equipment.

At this point, the reader should have a solid understanding of strength fitness, both in principle and practical application. Nonetheless, there are some relevant topics that were not covered in the text and others that merit additional attention. This chapter is designed to provide useful information in eleven of these related areas, and will answer questions on: (1) nutrition, (2) body composition, (3) muscle strength and endurance, (4) joint flexibility, (5) warm-ups and cool-downs, (6) female response, (7) over thirty response, (8) progress and assessment, (9) strength plateaus, (10) speed and performance power, and (11) bodybuilders and weightlifters.

Does Strength Training Require a Special Diet?

The questions most frequently asked by strength training enthusiasts are undoubtedly those related to diet, particularly the type and amount of protein that should be ingested for optimum muscular development. These are important questions, because proteins are partly responsible for the increased size and strength of trained muscle fibers. In addition to the actin and myosin proteins that form the structural and functional units of skeletal muscle, creatine protein is vital to the process of muscle contraction. Protein is also essential for the formation of bone tissue, blood, and the hormones that influence various physiological processes.

While few people question the importance of protein in the diet, there is considerable disagreement over the amount of protein one should consume on a daily basis, particularly when engaged in heavy strength training activities. The recommended daily protein requirement for adults is one gram of protein for every kilogram (2.2 pounds) of bodyweight. That is, an adult who weighs ninety kilograms (198 pounds) should obtain about ninety grams of protein, which is equivalent to 3.2 ounces of protein. Most Americans consume considerably more protein in the course of a day simply by following a normal, well-balanced diet. Persons who wish to increase their protein intake can easily do so by eating more protein-rich foods such as low-fat dairy products (milk, yogurt, and cottage cheese) and low-fat meats (chicken, turkey, fish, shellfish, and lean beef).

The fact is, however, that extra protein is not generally utilized by the body. With the possible exception of marathon runners, triathletes, and bodybuilders in heavy training, exercisers do not typically require additional protein if their daily diet is basically sound. This is true for most strength training participants, because the tissue building (anabolic) processes of the body occur at a relatively constant rate and are not significantly accelerated by the presence of additional protein. Consequently, excellent muscular development may be obtained without protein supplements if the exerciser adheres to sound nutritional guidelines.

Although there are numerous recommendations concerning training diets and nutritional supplements, there is no research evidence that a good basic diet can be improved upon in terms of enhancing one's muscular development. Such a diet provides the proteins, carbohydrates, fats, vitamins, minerals, and water necessary for optimum health. There are four basic categories of foods that should be included in one's daily meals.

Category 1: Meat-Poultry-Fish-Protein Foods

It is recommended that one obtain at least two servings per day of foods with a high protein content, such as the following:

Beans
Beef (lean)
Chicken
Egg whites
Fish
Lamb (lean)
Nuts (sparingly, due to high fat content)
Peanuts (sparingly, due to high fat content)
Pork (lean)
Shellfish
Soybeans (tofu) (sparingly, due to high fat content)
Turkey

Although it is not necessary to eat meat to achieve one's daily protein requirements, it is important to obtain all of the amino acids that are essential for protein synthesis. There are at least ten essential amino acids that cannot be manufactured in the human body and must be included in the diet. Meat, eggs, and milk products supply all of these essential amino acids, but no single vegetable, fruit, grain, or nut does so.

Because proteins obtained from animal sources contain all of the amino acids essential for tissue building and repair, they are often referred to as complete or high-quality proteins. Conversely, proteins derived from other food sources do not provide all of the essential amino acids, and are therefore called incomplete or low-quality proteins. It is possible for vegetarians to obtain all of the essential amino acids even though they do not consume meat or dairy products. They must, however, be knowledgeable about the types of proteins contained in their foods and be certain to eat a variety of vegetables, fruits, grains, and nuts to ensure that none of the essential amino acids are excluded from their diet.

Category 2: Dairy Products

In addition to the protein sources discussed in Category 1, it is recommended that one obtain two or more servings of dairy products on a daily basis. The following dairy products are excellent sources of high-quality proteins and calcium, which is an essential nutrient for muscle contraction and bone formation.

Cheese (hard)	Low-fat milk
Cottage cheese (low-fat)	Skim milk
Egg whites	Yogurt (low-fat)
Ice milk	

There has been considerable disagreement regarding the advantages and disadvantages of consuming dairy products when training for muscular strength and definition. The major point of controversy is over the relatively high-fat content of whole milk products. Because skim milk and other low-fat dairy products are readily available in nearly all grocery stores, there does not seem to be any good reason, other than allergic reactions, to avoid this highly nutritious food source. Skim milk furnishes the same amount of protein and calcium as whole milk but has less fat and fewer calories. It is interesting to note that the principal ingredient in most commercially prepared high-protein supplements (powders, pills, and liquids) is nonfat dried milk.

Category 3: Fruits and Vegetables

Fruits and vegetables should make up a large percentage of one's daily food intake. It is recommended that at least four servings from this group be consumed each day. All sorts of fruits and vegetables are included in this category, such as

Apples	Cauliflower	Onions
Asparagus	Celery	Peaches
Bananas	Cherries	Pears
Beans	Citrus fruits	Peas
Beets	Corn	Peppers
Berries	Dried fruits	Plums
Broccoli	Grapes	Potatoes
Cabbage	Lettuce	Squash
Carrots	Melons	Sweet potatoes
		Tomatoes

Although most fruits and vegetables do not have a high protein content, they are excellent sources for carbohydrates and the various vitamins and minerals that are necessary for physical health and peak performance.

Category 4: Cereals and Grains

Many Americans eat too few cereals and grains because they mistakenly believe these foods are high in fat. Actually, most foods in this group (breakfast cereal, bread, and pasta) have very little fat. Instead, they serve as excellent sources of complex carbohydrates, vitamins, and minerals, and reasonably good sources of protein. Consider the following food items that are made from cereals and grains:

Biscuits	Pancakes
Bran cereals	Pasta
Bread	Pastries
Corn cereals	Rice
Crackers	Rice cereals
Flour	Rolls
Muffins	Wheat cereals
Oat cereals	

Obviously, foods in this category may vary greatly in nutritional and caloric value. Basically, those that are highly refined and comprised largely of white flour, white sugar, and shortening are lower in nutritional value and higher in calories. Examples include cakes, cobblers, cookies, doughnuts, and pies. On the other hand, whole grain products such as dark breads, natural cereals, brown rice, and wheat germ have greater nutritional value and fewer calories. Other grain-based foods such as cereals, crackers, macaroni, and spaghetti fall somewhere in between, depending on the grain source utilized. Many grains and cereals have the additional advantage of providing fiber, which is important for efficient functioning of the digestive system.

Summary and Sample Diet for Bodybuilders

The person who eats a balanced diet (one that approximates the recommended number of servings from the four basic food groups) should obtain sufficient protein, as well as the necessary vitamins and minerals, to enable maximum gains in muscle size and strength.

In other words, protein supplementation is not necessary for promoting muscular gains. On the other hand, although excessive amounts of protein can place a burden on the kidneys, a small increase in one's protein consumption is not physically harmful and may be psychologically helpful to an athlete involved in heavy training. The author can think of few better ways to supplement one's diet, as long as a healthy balance among the four major food groups is maintained. Undoubtedly, a tuna fish sandwich, an apple, and a glass of skimmed milk provides a more nutritious lunch than a bag of potato chips, a candy bar, and a soft drink.

As indicated earlier in this section, proteins are composed of various combinations of amino acids. Because there are ten essential and ten nonessential amino acids, some protein foods are of more value than others in tissue building and repair. The best proteins for supplying human growth and maintenance needs are those from animal sources such as eggs, meat, fish, poultry, and milk products. However, because heavy consumption of meat appears to have a relatively high correlation with heart disease and certain types of cancer, it is recommended that several protein sources be utilized in the bodybuilder's diet.

Actually, meat ranks only sixth, behind eggs, milk, fish, cheese, and whole grain rice in terms of protein quality. Other sources of high-quality protein include oats, rye, wheat germ, wheat flour, soy flour, peas, beans, potatoes, and spinach. Various nuts, peanuts, and peanut butter are useful protein sources, but they also contain a high percentage of fat.

Of course, bodybuilders need foods from all of the basic food groups to meet their overall nutritional requirements. However, they typically ingest as little fat as possible to reduce subcutaneous fat deposits and enhance muscle definition.

With this in mind, a bodybuilder's breakfast might consist of whole wheat bread, wheat germ with raisins and low-fat milk, low-fat yogurt, and orange juice. For lunch, tuna packed in water, tossed salad with a tablespoon of oil and vinegar, low-fat milk, an apple, and an orange should suffice. The evening meal could include broiled fish with lemon, whole grain rice, sweet potatoes, peas, rye bread without butter, fresh fruit salad, vegetable juice, low-fat milk, and walnut-stuffed dates. Appropriate snack foods could include low-fat yogurt, low-fat milk, fresh fruit, raisins, dates, and cereals.

The sample menu is presented simply as a guideline for obtaining good nutrition while emphasizing high-quality protein consumption and restricting fat intake. It should go without saying that chicken, turkey, lean beef, or veal could be substituted for fish and that a wide variety of fruits, vegetables, whole grains, and low-fat dairy products could be interchanged without disrupting the basic concept of the bodybuilder's diet.

How Does Strength Training Affect Body Composition?

There has been a widespread misunderstanding regarding the relationship between muscle and fat, particularly with respect to weight training. It is often said that the muscle one develops during the training period will turn to fat once the program is discontinued. This sometimes appears to be the case but actually cannot happen. Muscle is a tissue that tends to get larger when it is used (hypertrophy) and smaller when it is not used (atrophy). Fat is a substance that accumulates in various parts of the body when one's caloric intake exceeds one's energy expenditure. Muscle cannot physically become fat or vice versa.

What frequently happens is this. A person begins a strength training program and experiences muscle hypertrophy. During the training period, caloric intake is increased to meet the new energy and tissue-building requirements of the body. Because the energy demand is equal to the energy supply, fat is not deposited, and the exerciser displays a well-defined muscular physique. Then, when for some reason the strength training program is discontinued, the muscles begin to decrease in size (atrophy). If the caloric intake is not correspondingly reduced to equal the lower energy requirements, fat will begin to accumulate. Consequently, the muscle may be replaced by fat as a result of stopping the exercise program but maintaining the same eating behavior. This phenomenon can be avoided by adjusting one's diet to the level of activity or inactivity. When this is done, the individual who stops working out will experience a gradual loss of muscle size and body weight, but will not become fat.

Another misconception concerning weight training is that the training process inevitably makes one bulky. The truth is that many weightlifters are bulky to begin with, not because they train with weights. For example, a stocky boy or girl may find little success in sports requiring speed, endurance, or agility and may turn to weight training as an alternative activity. The weight training will increase muscle size and strength, but will not, by itself, eliminate a bulky appearance. Only a proper combination of diet and vigorous exercise can produce such a slimming effect. Consequently, one should not assume that a bulky weightlifter looks that way because of the strength training program. More than likely, he or she retains that appearance in spite of the strength training program.

It should be understood that one's basic body build cannot be substantially changed by a weight training program. There is no evidence that strength training can alter skeletal structure or increase the length of one's muscle bellies. Even the degree to which one gains muscle strength and size is genetically determined and regulated through hormone production.

In other words, strength training is limited in application to the muscles being exercised. One can bulk up by lifting weights and overeating, and one can slim down by lifting weights and under-eating, but large changes in body weight are more likely the result of eating patterns than strength training programs.

If one is concerned with both losing fat and building muscle, then strength training is the ideal activity. Although aerobic activity (e.g., running, cycling, and swimming) burns many calories, it does not increase muscle mass. These activities have a single reducing effect, because they only burn calories while they are being performed (and for a short recovery period following the exercise session).

On the other hand, strength training burns calories and increases muscle mass. Because greater muscle mass requires greater energy supplies, strength training has a double reducing effect. That is, strength training burns calories during the exercise session and during the rest of the day due to the higher metabolic needs of larger muscles.

This is not to suggest that aerobic activities are less important. Aerobic conditioning is fundamental to physical fitness. However, strength training should be included in fat-loss programs. One study (Westcott 1987b) found that dieting with aerobic exercise resulted in both fat loss and muscle loss, whereas dieting with aerobic exercise and strength exercise produced simultaneous fat loss and muscle gain.

The combination program (diet, aerobic exercise, and strength exercise) is recommended because it has a better effect on body composition and metabolic rate.

It is suggested that one follow five guidelines to lose fat in a safe and sensible manner. First, one should eat three to four moderate-sized meals per day. Second, one should reduce fat intake to less than 25 percent of the daily caloric consumption. Third, one should reduce daily caloric consumption by 10 percent. Actually, reducing fat intake automatically decreases caloric intake because fats have twice as many calories per gram as proteins and carbohydrates. Fourth, one should perform regular strength training to use more calories and to increase muscle mass. Three twenty-minute strength training sessions per week are recommended. Fifth, one should perform regular endurance training to burn additional calories and to improve cardiovascular fitness. Three twenty-minute aerobic sessions per week are sufficient, although daily aerobic activity may be preferred.

Does Muscle Strength Affect Muscle Endurance?

As discussed in chapter 4, some people have low-endurance muscles and others have high-endurance muscles. However, the relationship between one's muscle strength and relative muscle endurance is apparently fixed due to genetic factors. For example, most individuals can complete about ten repetitions with 75 percent of their maximum resistance. Therefore, if Jim is able to squat 100 pounds once, he can probably perform ten repetitions with 75 pounds. If he increases his maximum squat to 200 pounds, he should complete ten repetitions with 150 pounds. In other words, regardless of his strength level, he will always lift 75 percent of his maximum resistance about ten times.

Conversely, Jim's absolute muscle endurance automatically increases as his strength increases. When Jim's maximum squat was 100 pounds, he could perform ten repetitions with the 75-pound weightload. When Jim's maximum squat reaches 200 pounds he should complete many more repetitions with the 75-pound weightload because that resistance is now a much smaller percentage (37.5 percent) of his maximum.

Table 8.1   Bench press training program

Week	Monday	Wednesday	Friday
1	45 lb. × 5	45 lb. × 5	50 lb. × 5
2	50 lb. × 5	55 lb. × 3	55 lb. × 3
3	55 lb. × 4	55 lb. × 5	55 lb. × 5
4	60 lb. × 2	60 lb. × 2	60 lb. × 2
5	60 lb. × 2	60 lb. × 3	60 lb. × 4
6	60 lb. × 5	60 lb. × 5	Test day

Table 8.2   Performance tests in bench press exercise before and after six-week training program

Bench press exercise	Before training	After training	Percent increase
Maximum Weightload	55 lbs.	70 lbs.	27%
Repetitions Completed with 25 lbs.	36 reps.	52 reps.	44%

Consider the results of a research study the author conducted on his wife during the summer of 1976 as part of his doctoral studies. Using the bench press exercise, she was tested for her maximum weightload. She was also tested for the number of repetitions she could complete with 45 percent of her maximum weightload. The training protocol consisted of one set of bench presses, three days per week (see table 8.1). After six weeks of training, she was again tested for her maximum weightload and the number of repetitions she could complete with 45 percent of her original maximum weightload. As shown in table 8.2, her maximum weightload increased from fifty-five to seventy pounds. This represented a 27 percent increase in muscle strength. Her performance with twenty-five pounds (45 percent of her original maximum weightload) increased from thirty-six to fifty-two repetitions. This represented a 44 percent increase in muscle endurance with a specific weightload.

Although the training program was strictly strength oriented, lasting no longer than thirty seconds per session, the subject experienced a 44 percent improvement in absolute muscle endurance. This result supports a strong positive relationship between muscle strength and muscle endurance.

From a practical perspective, it would not seem necessary to train for both muscle strength and muscle endurance. It would appear that one automatically increases absolute muscle endurance as one increases muscle strength. As the given resistance becomes a lower percentage of the new maximum resistance it is simply easier to perform.

How Does Strength Training Affect Joint Flexibility

Flexibility refers to the range of motion in a joint, and has an important relationship to injury prevention and force production. Although an optimum range of joint movement has not been established, a restricted movement range increases the likelihood of injury. Also, joint mobility is an important factor in athletic performance. For example, the greater the distance over which an object is accelerated, the greater the force produced. Consequently, a discus thrower who increases shoulder girdle flexibility will throw farther if all other factors remain the same.

The key to joint flexibility is muscle stretchability. Muscle stretchability is best accomplished through full-range movements with a significant pause in the fully stretched position. Muscles possess a property referred to as elasticity. That is, they return to their normal resting length after being stretched. However, if the stretch is sudden, specialized control mechanisms called muscle spindles initiate a stretch reflex that produces a rapid and forceful muscle contraction. This is a protective reaction to prevent the muscle from being damaged by an abrupt or uncontrolled stretching force. For this reason, stretching exercises should never be performed quickly.

Many people develop a specific stretching program to enhance their joint flexibility. However, properly executed strength training is also an effective means for improving flexibility. For example, when the biceps muscle is completely contracted, the triceps muscle is fully stretched. Likewise, when the triceps muscle is completely contracted, the biceps muscle is fully stretched. Consequently, if one trains all of the major muscle groups, one will also stretch all of the major muscle groups. The slow movements that are best for muscle strengthening are also best for muscle stretching.

It should be understood that muscle strength and muscle stretchability are different qualities. The former represents a muscle's ability to contract, and the latter represents a muscle's ability to relax. Neither ability has great influence on the other. A high level of strength does not prevent a high level of flexibility, or vice versa. An exerciser can develop both strength and flexibility through a well-designed and properly executed strength training program.

How Important Are Warm-Ups and Cool-Downs?

There has been considerable controversy over the advantages, disadvantages, or neutrality of performing warm-up exercises prior to athletic events and strenuous exercise sessions. Those in favor of using warm-ups generally believe that the resulting increase in body temperature enhances the physical performance that follows. Those not in favor of warming up counter that increased body temperature is one of the factors that limits athletic performance, particularly in endurance-type activities. In either case, it is interesting to note that most warm-up routines have a rather limited effect on muscle temperature.

With regard to muscle stretchability, most people can temporarily increase their range of movement after performing stretching exercises. Some people prefer to stretch prior to the activity, while others feel that stretching is more useful immediately following the activity. If range of movement is an important performance factor, appropriate stretching exercises should probably be done during the warm-up.

Activities that require precise movement patterns seem to benefit from prior rehearsal in the form of progressively more forceful trials. For example, baseball pitchers, football quarterbacks, and shot putters invariably warm up with a few easy throws, then gradually increase their intensity until they are throwing at full effort. While this procedure seems to help groove the desired response pattern for movements that require fine motor control, its effect on the performance of gross motor movements, such as most weight training exercises, is not known.

Competitive weightlifters may perform progressively heavier sets in some of their training exercises. This may be both physiologically beneficial in preparing the muscles for heavier weightloads, and serve as a psychological aid for building the exerciser's confidence prior to the big lifts.

On the other hand, if the exercise set consists of ten repetitions, it is probably not necessary to perform preliminary warm-up sets with lighter weights. Under normal circumstances, a weightload that can be lifted ten times should not cause injury or require special preparation. For example, if Alan can complete ten leg extensions in good form with 100 pounds he is training safely with about 75 percent of his maximum weightload (see chapter 4). If each repetition requires seven seconds, Alan will take almost one minute to perform the first eight repetitions. During this time, the quadriceps muscles experience a specific warm-up, and are well prepared for the final two repetitions. In other words, by the time the quadriceps muscles exert maximum effort, they have had sixty seconds of progressively more difficult repetitions to stimulate the appropriate physiological adjustments. Nonetheless, it is probably a good practice to perform a few minutes of continuous large muscle activity prior to strength training as an added safety precaution. According to Westcott's (1986g) research, twenty minutes of cycling prior to the strength training workout did not significantly reduce muscle performance.

Although more attention is generally given to the warm-up process, the cool-down period that follows the workout is very important. Because strength training is a high-intensity activity, large amounts of energy must be supplied to the muscles during contraction. Assuming that most exercise sets take about seventy seconds, part of this energy is supplied through anaerobic glycolysis and produces a fatigue by-product known as lactic acid. The process of energy replacement and lactic acid removal may be affected by one's post exercise activity. The person who completes the exercise session with ten to fifteen minutes of moderate activity (walking, jogging, or swimming) is likely to experience a faster recovery rate.

The most critical aspect of the cool-down is to facilitate blood return to the heart. If one simply stops exercising, blood tends to accumulate in the extremities, placing considerable stress on the heart and circulatory system. By continuing to exercise at a lower intensity, rhythmic muscle contractions assist blood flow and permit a gradual return to resting circulation.

To be most effective, the cool-down should conclude with some muscle stretching exercises. In a very real sense, the cool-down may mean the difference between leaving the locker room feeling exhausted or feeling invigorated.

How Do Women Respond to Strength Training?

The average American woman is approximately four inches shorter and thirty pounds lighter than the average American man. In addition, she has about fifteen pounds more fat weight and about forty-five pounds less lean body weight (e.g., muscle, bone, and organs). It is therefore not surprising that most females are weaker than their male counterparts. Indeed, strength assessments reveal that males typically use twice as much weight in upper body exercises and 50 percent more weight in lower body exercises (Westcott, Benkis, and McPhee 1985).

More specifically, muscle tissue can produce a certain amount of contractile force per square centimeter of size, regardless of gender. Therefore, the concept that a larger muscle is a stronger muscle applies to both males and females. However, due to genetic factors and hormone differences, men typically start with larger muscles and develop greater muscle hypertrophy than women.

Women will increase muscle mass to some degree as a result of strength training, but changes in body size are difficult to predict. For example, in one study (Westcott 1984a) previously untrained women increased their arm girth by ¼ inch after one month of strength training. In another study (Westcott 1988k) previously untrained women decreased their arm girth by ½ inch after two months of strength training. In the first study, the subjects' increase in arm girth represented more muscle gain than fat loss in this body part. In the second study, the subjects' decrease in arm girth represented more fat loss than muscle gain in this body part.

Although women rarely develop large muscles, they can certainly develop strong muscles. In fact, due to their lower initial strength, females may gain strength at a faster rate than males. Westcott (1986j) noted that identical strength training programs produced a 40 percent performance improvement in male subjects and a 70 percent performance improvement in female subjects over the course of the training period.

Also, as discussed in chapter 3, women can develop lower body strength that compares favorably to men on a pound-for-pound basis. In a strength assessment of 900 adults, Westcott (1986i) found that the average male could perform ten strict leg extensions with 62 percent of his bodyweight, while the average female could complete ten strict leg extensions with 55 percent of her bodyweight.

It is important to understand that women can improve their muscle strength and physical appearance through a progressive program of strength training. The only training response difference between men and women is the degree to which muscle strength and hypertrophy are developed. The strength training principles and procedures are identical for males and females, and the same basic exercise program is effective for men and women.

How Do Persons Over Thirty Respond to Strength Training?

Persons over thirty respond to strength training almost the same as persons under thirty. The only difference is the rate of strength gain. During the first two decades of life, the body undergoes muscle growth and development due to normal maturation processes. After reaching adulthood, the person who does not perform regular strength training experiences a gradual decrease in muscle strength. The rate of strength loss becomes greater during the succeeding decades and is a natural consequence of the aging process. In addition to strength decrement, growing older is accompanied by a decrease in metabolic rate and a reduction in maximum heart rate. Properly performed strength training has a positive influence on the first two degenerative processes. Through progressive resistance exercise, men and women can achieve and maintain relatively high strength levels during their thirties, forties, fifties, and sixties. Because there is a direct relationship between strong muscles and strong bones, strength training may be particularly useful for older men and women who are subject to bone loss.

Another benefit of strength training is increased muscle mass. In addition to producing firmer muscles, this results in a higher metabolic rate due to the increased energy requirements of larger muscles. As discussed in chapter 4, every pound of muscle that one develops requires additional calories throughout the day for tissue maintenance and repair functions.

With the exception of those who have continued to train during adulthood, one's current strength level can be increased regardless of age. That is, adults who begin a strength training program will experience gains in muscular strength whether they are thirty-five or sixty-five, and the improved muscle fitness will help them to look better, feel better, and function better.

As a hypothetical example, let's assume that Mr. Jones was an avid weightlifter during his college years, and at that time was capable of bench pressing 300 pounds. After graduation, he discontinued his training program and has done nothing more strenuous than lawn work and recreational sports for the past twenty years. Now, at forty years of age, he decides to engage in serious strength training once again. He finds that, although he is about 15 pounds heavier than his college weight, he can now bench press only 160 pounds. After four months of training he is able to bench press 220 pounds, and after one year he is up to 270 pounds. Further training maintains but does not increase his strength level. In comparison to his college best, Mr. Jones is only 90 percent (270 lbs./300 lbs.) as strong at forty-one years of age as he was at age twenty. However, he is 170 percent (270 lbs./160 lbs.) stronger at forty-one years of age than he was at forty, and much more fit.

Weight training has been accused of causing damage to the heart and circulatory system due to its strenuous nature. Actually, research indicates that sensible strength training may actually improve cardiovascular function and reduce resting blood pressure (see chapter 4). Sensible strength training is characterized by continuous movement and continuous breathing throughout each exercise set. Holding the breath or holding the weight in a static position for more than a moment may occlude blood flow and elevate blood pressure. While these guidelines should be followed by all exercisers, they are a must for persons over thirty years of age and for persons who have coronary risk factors.

Whenever the exerciser reaches a sticking point, the set should be terminated and the weight immediately lowered. Prolonged straining to complete a final repetition is not necessary for strength development and is a potentially dangerous procedure for persons with circulatory problems. With respect to overexertion, weight training may be compared to snow shoveling. Persons who work within their capacity, lifting reasonable loads of snow, should not experience any difficulty in clearing the driveway. On the other hand, persons who struggle to carry as much snow as possible every time they lift the shovel may be headed for trouble.

Because weight training permits a wide range of resistance, it is an excellent strength building activity for persons of all ages. No matter how weak a person may be, the weightload may be adjusted so that ten repetitions can be completed with appropriate effort. This is not always the case for other strength-related exercises, such as pull-ups, in which only one or two repetitions may be possible.

It is recommended that persons over 30 follow a basic strength training program. They should exercise each of the major muscle groups and observe the standard training principles and procedures presented in chapter 5. Although the adult who has not been physically active should have a medical checkup before beginning a vigorous exercise program, it has been aptly stated that a medical examination is perhaps more necessary for the adult who chooses to remain sedentary.

What About Progress and Assessment?

The development of strength fitness is a complex phenomenon that involves numerous physiological adaptations to imposed training stimuli. Persons who effectively apply the principles of stress adaptation, rebuilding time, near-maximum resistance, movement speed, movement range, muscle balance, and continuous breathing generally enjoy a safe and productive training experience. Sensible strength training typically results in a high rate of strength gain and a low incidence of tissue injury.

Although the relationship between strength training and strength improvement is relatively stable over time, it is somewhat unpredictable on a day-to-day or week-to-week basis. For example, table 8.3 presents the rates of strength gain over successive 2½ week training periods for three different groups of college males (Westcott 1974). Group A made the greatest strength increment during the first 2½-week training period. Group B experienced the highest strength increase during the second 2½-week training period, and Group C achieved the greatest strength gain during the third 2½-week training interval.

Generally speaking, as one continues to train, greater stimulus is required to produce further strength gains. That is, more training stress is necessary to maintain one's muscular progress. A problem arises, however, when greater and greater amounts of stress result in smaller and smaller increments in strength. This state of affairs, often referred to as staleness, is common to athletes in all fitness-related activities. Distance runners and weightlifters are alike in that improvement comes more quickly during the first weeks of practice

Table 8.3 Rates of strength gain over successive 2½ week training periods for three different training groups

Training group	Number	Average strength increase during first 2½ weeks of training	Average strength increase during second 2½ weeks of training	Average strength increase during third 2½ weeks of training
A	13	10.6%	6.1%	5.4%
B	20	5.5%	5.7%	4.6%
C	16	6.4%	4.0%	7.2%

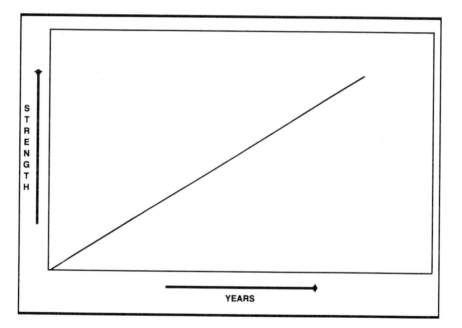

Figure 8.1 Hypothetical relationship between strength development and years of training. In this example, the rate of strength gain remains constant throughout the duration of the training program.

and less easily as they get closer to their maximum performance potential. For example, a weightlifter who increases his bench press by five pounds a week at the start of his program may improve less than five pounds a year after several years of training, even though the training intensity is considerably greater.

Although it would be nice if everyone's rate of strength gain resembled that displayed in figure 8.1, a more accurate and realistic representation of strength development is presented in figure 8.2. As

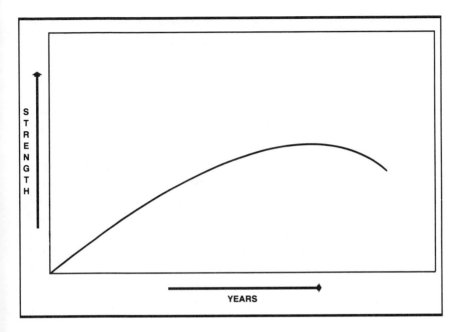

Figure 8.2 Hypothetical relationship between strength development and years of training. In this example, the rate of strength gain decreases throughout the duration of the training program, and eventually becomes a rate of strength loss.

indicated in the latter figure, the rate of strength gain decreases throughout the duration of one's training career and eventually becomes a rate of strength decrement due to the aging process. The nontraining individual begins to lose strength after age twenty, but the person who trains can maintain strength for many more years and postpone the strength loss that eventually accompanies middle age.

Basically, the principle of diminishing returns applies to the process of strength development. At first, brief workouts result in relatively large strength gains. Later, long workouts produce relatively small increments in strength. For years, weightlifters have rebelled against diminishing rates of strength development by doubling and tripling the length of their training sessions. It is doubtful that this practice significantly increases their rate of strength gain, and may actually produce the opposite effect. At best, too much stress prevents positive strength adaptations. At worst, it results in chronically fatigued muscles, strength decrement, and tissue injury.

Well-informed exercisers realize that strength gains come more slowly as training continues. They do not fight this natural phenomenon, but simply train in harmony with it. They do not expend double the time and energy necessary to achieve optimum improvement. Instead, they periodically change the training variables in a systematic attempt to stimulate further strength development. There are essentially five training variables that may be altered: (1) the training exercises, (2) the training frequency, (3) the training sets, (4) the repetitions-resistance relationships, and (5) the training intensity.

The key to continued progress is gradual improvement and sensitivity to potential stumbling blocks. The strength training logbook is an invaluable tool for assessing progress and for correcting small problems before they become major obstacles to strength development. The training logbook should include the date and time of the workout. It should also specify the exercise, the weightload, the repetitions, and any notations such as seat height or technique adaptations. A sample strength training logbook is presented in Appendix E.

The training logbook provides a systematic means for comparing you to yourself, and that is the only meaningful comparison to make. Comparisons with beginners are usually discouraging because beginners tend to have higher rates of strength gain. Comparisons with advanced trainers are equally discouraging because these individuals have typically attained higher strength levels.

One means of assessing progress is to ask the question, "How does my training today compare with my training four weeks ago?" For such comparison to be meaningful, there must be a degree of consistency in one's training program over a period of time. This is not to suggest that people should never alter a training routine, but that they should stay with a given exercise program long enough for it to be effective. As a rule of thumb, a specific training program should be given a four-week trial period to fairly assess its impact on strength development.

Continued progress is dependent upon the identification and incorporation of those training procedures that are most effective for producing strength gains. People who train on a day-to-day basis are less likely to have positive exercise experiences than those who take a programmatic approach to strength development.

How Can One Avoid Strength Plateaus?

When progress comes to a halt, one is said to be on a strength plateau. Generally speaking, a strength plateau indicates some aspect of the training program should be altered. As noted in the previous section, such a change usually involves one or more of the following training variables: (1) exercise selection, (2) exercise frequency, (3) exercise sets, (4) repetitions-resistance relationships, and (5) exercise intensity.

Although there may be numerous training considerations (including equipment, rest, diet, partners, etc.), the basic decision is whether to make one's workout more demanding or less demanding. It has been the author's experience that persons on a strength plateau often choose to work harder in an attempt to force further strength development. In many cases, this strategy either maintains the plateau level of strength or results in strength loss. Doing more of the same activity that led to the strength plateau seldom initiates new strength gains. The better alternative is to examine one's workout program and make constructive changes to stimulate new muscle growth.

Exercise Selection

The first step may be a change in the training exercises. For example, if progress has come to a halt in the bench press exercise, it might be beneficial to substitute weighted bar dips. While both exercises utilize the same muscle groups (pectoralis major, anterior deltoid, and triceps), the movement patterns elicit different neuromuscular responses. This results in a new order of muscle fiber recruitment that can stimulate further improvement in both exercise performance and muscle development. Research indicates that the motor learning factors associated with new exercises may play a major role in overcoming strength plateaus (see chapter 4). As presented in chapter 7, there are several exercises that can be performed for each of the major muscle groups.

Exercise Frequency

The second consideration has to do with the exercise frequency. Sometimes it is helpful to reduce one's workout demands temporarily to allow the muscle recovery and rebuilding process to catch up. Remember that positive muscle adaptations occur during the rest periods following the training sessions. Consequently, it may be beneficial to schedule more time between successive workouts.

Exercise Sets

A third alternative, for exercisers who prefer multiple set training, is to increase or decrease the number of sets performed. On the one hand, trainers who complete ten to fifteen sets per body part should ask themselves how much advantage or disadvantage they experience by continuing to work a muscle group after it has been thoroughly stressed. On the other hand, persons involved in pyramid training programs may benefit from several progressively heavier lead-up sets. As a rule of thumb, the more exercises performed, the fewer sets. For those who have difficulty maintaining a high level of exercise intensity throughout the workout, single set training may be preferable.

Repetitions-Resistance Relationships

Another area that should be examined is the repetitions-resistance relationships. It may be helpful to perform more repetitions at a lower resistance or to execute fewer repetitions at a higher resistance. For example, the quadriceps muscles may be so accustomed to performing twelve repetitions with 140 pounds that this training protocol no longer promotes positive strength adaptations. If this is the case, switching to eight repetitions with 160 pounds may stimulate the quadriceps to be more responsive. Frequent variations in the repetitions-resistance relationship seems to be an effective means for reducing both physical and mental staleness.

Exercise Intensity

Breakdown Training

It is also possible that the exercise intensity must be increased for further strength development. As discussed in chapter 5, breakdown training represents an effective means for fatiguing additional muscle fibers following an exhaustive exercise bout. Generally speaking, when one completes ten repetitions with 75 percent of maximum resistance, 25 percent of the muscle fibers reach failure. If the resistance is immediately reduced a small amount, the exerciser can perform a few more repetitions by recruiting additional muscle fibers. By so doing he has gone to failure twice, and forcefully fatigued more muscle fibers during the extended set of high-effort exercise.

Assisted Training

Another technique, known as assisted training, accomplishes the same objective with the help of a training partner. Instead of reducing the resistance at the point of muscle failure, a training partner manually assists the exerciser with a few more repetitions. A skillful training partner enables the exerciser to forcefully fatigue more muscle fibers during the extended set of high-effort exercise.

Negative Training

A third form of high intensity training emphasizes the negative or eccentric phase of strength exercise. Because eccentric contractions are capable of producing over 40 percent more force than concentric contractions, it may be possible to increase the strength stimulus by stressing the negative (lowering) movements. Unfortunately, negative training may also increase the risk of tissue injury. It is therefore extremely important to perform negative training in a slow and controlled manner.

One type of negative training involves a partner who helps lift a heavier weight than the exerciser can handle. The exerciser then lowers the weight slowly by means of forceful eccentric contractions.

Another means of negative training is performing as many positive repetitions as possible, then receiving assistance on a few additional lifting movements while working hard on the lowering movements (assisted training).

Negative training may also be helpful for improving performance in bodyweight exercises such as pull-ups and bar dips. Persons who are not strong enough to lift their bodyweight can climb to the top position and lower themselves slowly. The same muscles used concentrically to lift the body are used eccentrically to lower the body.

Super-Slow Training

Perhaps the safest form of high-intensity exercise is known as super-slow training. Super-slow training is generally characterized by a ten-second lifting movement, a momentary pause in the fully contracted position, and a four-second lowering movement. As each repetition requires about fifteen seconds, four to six repetitions are usually sufficient. In fact, because there is almost no momentum, sixty to ninety seconds of super-slow training is very demanding physically and provides an excellent stimulus for strength development.

Super-Set Training

Super-set training refers to two successive exercises for the same body part. For example, immediately following a set of lat pulldowns one may perform a set of low rows. Both exercises involve the latissimus dorsi, upper back, posterior deltoids, and biceps, but in a different movement pattern. Super-set training forces the target muscle groups to perform double duty. However, because the exact exercise movement is not duplicated, the muscle fiber recruitment pattern is somewhat different and the training stimulus is enhanced.

Strength plateaus appear to be an inevitable consequence of continued training. Regardless of the training program utilized, there comes a time when a change of one type or another seems necessary to stimulate further strength development. Strength plateaus should not be cause for discouragement. They are simply reminders that it is time to revise the training routine. It may be an indication for new exercises, more rest, fewer sets, different repetitions-resistance relationships, or higher intensity training. Whatever changes may be indicated, they should be viewed as positive steps toward one's optimum muscular development.

Can Strength Training Improve Speed and Performance Power?

Speed

Speed is an important factor for successful performance in many athletic activities. Most sports participants would like to increase their speed of movement (running speed, throwing speed, striking speed, kicking speed, etc.) to enhance their performance level. Unfortunately, as every track coach knows, it is not easy to improve one's movement speed.

Speed is a complex neuromuscular phenomenon. Basically speaking, some people have it and some people do not. Although speed can be improved, no one really knows the best means for doing so. It is generally agreed that speed is most likely to be developed through repeated practice efforts. According to physiologists, high-quality repetition of a sports skill increases the probability that the more efficient nerve pathways will become grooved, and that the less efficient nerve pathways will be avoided.

Speed training should be performed as quickly as possible to produce the desired results. Because added resistance automatically slows movement time, strength training may not be a very effective means for enhancing one's movement speed. For example, let's say that a soccer player wants to increase the speed of her instep kick. She decides to do quick repetitions with fifty pounds in the leg extension exercise. Unfortunately, she cannot move a fifty-pound resistance nearly as fast as she can kick a soccer ball. Consequently, it is doubtful that this type of training will produce a faster instep kicking action.

Performance Power

Speed and power are often spoken of interchangeably, but they actually represent different physical capacities. In fact, speed is one component of power. With respect to the human body, performance power is the product of movement speed and muscle force.

$$\text{Performance Power} = \text{Movement Speed} \times \text{Muscle Force}$$

In accordance with this formula, one may improve performance by increasing the movement speed component, increasing the muscle force component, or both. As presented in chapter 5, this may be more difficult than it appears because there is an optimum combination of movement speed and muscle force necessary for maximum power production. Too much speed reduces the muscle force component and too little speed reduces the movement speed component.

It is therefore the author's opinion that one perform high-quality skill training to improve movement speed and high-intensity strength training to improve muscle force.

Because skill training is highly specific to each athletic event, this topic will not be addressed. Muscle force, however, may be generally improved by applying the principles of sensible strength training. Other things being equal, as one develops greater muscle force he or she should demonstrate greater performance power.

Over the past several years, coaches have learned that weight training can increase muscle size and strength without reducing speed and flexibility. Most athletic coaches, therefore, include some form of strength training in their sports programs. Athletes involved in team sports (e.g., football, soccer, basketball, volleyball, baseball, softball, lacrosse, hockey, and European handball), dual sports (e.g., tennis, badminton, racquetball, handball, and wrestling) and individual sports (e.g., track and field, cross-country, swimming and diving, gymnastics, bicycling, canoeing, golf, and archery) can all benefit from well-designed strength training programs.

Although some people are interested in specific strength training exercises for various sports, it should be understood that the main purpose of strength training is to increase muscle strength. Strength exercises that simulate specific sports skills may be more harmful than helpful, and should be approached with caution.

For example, some athletes perform simulated throwing movements with added resistance. This is unlikely to increase their throwing speed, as added resistance always results in slower movement speeds. Also, performing throwing movements with added resistance places considerable stress on the shoulder, elbow, and wrist joints, and may cause tissue injury. Finally, the added resistance is usually insufficient to stimulate significant gains in strength.

For these reasons, the author's preferred means for developing muscle force is a standard strength training program. As athletes learn how to utilize their increased muscle force through quality skill practice, they should experience noticeable improvement in performance power.

What Is the Difference between Bodybuilders and Weightlifters?

Certain individuals possess the genetic potential to develop unusually large and strong muscles. With appropriate training, such men and women can become successful bodybuilders or weightlifters (Olympic lifts and power lifts). Although there are some similarities between bodybuilders and weightlifters, there are many essential differences.

Bodybuilders are more concerned with the internal response of the muscles, whereas weightlifters are more concerned with the external response of the barbell. Bodybuilders direct their training efforts toward increasing muscle size, and typically appear stronger than they are. Weightlifters, on the other hand, direct their training efforts toward increasing muscle strength, and are generally stronger than they appear.

While there is a definite relationship between muscle size and muscle strength, at the competitive level training programs are highly specialized. The most striking difference between bodybuilders and weightlifters is the amount of rest they take between successive sets of exercise.

Bodybuilders take very short rest periods (fifteen to forty-five seconds) between sets in order to "pump" their muscles. The muscle pump represents a temporary increase in muscle size due to the accumulation of blood. Quickly repeated bouts of exercise maintain fluid congestion in the target muscle area and produce the pumped up feeling. Because brief rest periods permit only partial recovery, bodybuilders train with relatively low percentages of their maximum resistance. For example, a bodybuilder who can bench press 300 pounds may perform six sets of ten reps with 200 pounds during a typical training session. Due to brief recovery periods, he is forced to work with about 65 percent of his maximum resistance.

Conversely, weightlifters take rather long rest periods (three to six minutes) between sets in order to recover as much strength as possible for each lifting bout. Because weightlifters must practice with relatively high percentages of their maximum resistance, more complete recovery is necessary between training sets. For example, a powerlifter who can bench press 300 pounds may perform the following pyramid workout with four to five minute rests between sets.

$$160 \times 10 \qquad 190 \times 8 \qquad 220 \times 6 \qquad 250 \times 4$$
$$280 \times 2 \qquad 280 \times 2 \qquad 280 \times 2$$

As a result of long recovery periods, he can train with almost 95 percent of his maximum resistance.

Table 8.4 presents representative training protocols for competitive bodybuilders and weightlifters. It should be noted that due to genetic factors, bodybuilders and weightlifters appear to have two distinct training advantages. First, they seem to endure highly stressful workouts with less risk of injury than the average person. Second, they typically respond to muscle training stimuli with greater size (hypertrophy) and strength gains than the average individual.

This is not to say that bodybuilders and weightlifters do not experience injuries, nor that they do not train long and hard. They do. It is to suggest that persons who do not possess favorable genetic characteristics for these sports refrain from following the champions' advanced training programs. These demanding exercise protocols are much too stressful for the average strength trainer, and generally lead to overuse injuries. Persons interested in pursuing bodybuilding or weightlifting should find a competent coach, and train systematically toward progressive competitive goals.

Table 8.4   Representative training protocol for bodybuilders and weightlifters

	Bodybuilders (muscle size)	Weightlifters (muscle strength)
Exercises	3–5 per muscle group	1–2 per muscle group
Sets	4–6 per exercise	6–8 per exercise
Resistance	65%–75% maximum	80%–95% maximum
Repetitions	10–15 per set	2–8 per set
Rest between sets	15–45 seconds	3–6 minutes

Appendix A

Strength Training Equipment

Further information regarding strength training equipment can be obtained by contacting the following manufacturers:

Cybex Eagle
2100 Smithtown Ave.
P.O. Box 9003
Ronkonkoma, NY 11779-0903

Hammer Strength
P.O. Box 19040
Cincinnati, OH 45219

Hydra Fitness Industries
P.O. Box 599
Belton, TX 76513-0599

Keiser Sports Health Equipment
411 S. West Ave.
Fresno, CA 93706-9952

Nautilus Sports Medical Industries
P.O. Box 809014
Dallas, TX 75380-9014

Universal Gym
Nissen-Universal
P.O. Box 1270
Cedar Rapids, IA 52406

Weider Barbell Company
21100 Erwin Street
Woodland Hills, CA 91367

York Barbell Company
P.O. Box 1707
York, PA 17405

Appendix B

Principles of Force Production

There are certain basic principles of movement that should be observed when attempting to impart force to an object. The following principles of force production should be understood and applied by athletes involved in dynamic sports events.

Production of Force: To apply maximum force to an object, engage the maximum number of contributing muscle groups.

Direction of Force: To apply maximum force to an object, direct the force through the center of mass of the body and of the object.

Summation of Force: To apply maximum force to an object, begin each successive force at the height of the previous force.

Transfer of Weight: To apply maximum force to an object, move the center of mass in the direction of the force.

Range of Movement: To apply maximum force to an object, accelerate the object over the maximum possible distance.

Speed of Movement: To apply maximum force to an object, accelerate the object in the shortest possible time.

Action-Reaction: To apply maximum force to an object, maintain contact with the ground while the object is being accelerated.

Stretch Reaction: To develop maximum force, precede each muscular contraction with an initial stretch.

Absorption of Force: To absorb an impact, spread the force over the maximum area and the maximum distance possible.

Appendix C

Training Effects of Endurance Exercise

Research during the last several years has clearly demonstrated that regular physical exercise of sufficient intensity and duration can produce remarkable adaptations in the cardiovascular system. Beneficial physiological changes take place in the heart, the blood vessels, the blood itself, and the musculoskeletal system. There appears to be an all-or-none law that triggers these internal developments. The three components neccessary for cardiovascular improvement are: (1) an exercise intensity sufficient to raise the heart rate to approximately 70 percent of maximum, (2) an exercise duration of at least fifteen to twenty minutes and preferably longer, (3) an exercise frequency of at least three nonconsecutive days per week and preferably more often. Although any physical activity that meets these criteria is acceptable, those that are rhythmical and easily controlled (e.g., walking, jogging, bicycling, stationary bicycling, swimming, and rope jumping) seem most useful for promoting cardiovascular fitness.

What follows is a partial list of the training effects of an endurance exercise program. In addition to the incredible adaptations exhibited by the cardiovascular system, it is interesting to note that the untrained heart may contract about 40,000 more times per day than the trained heart in order to circulate the same blood volume.

Training Effects

I. Heart becomes a stronger pump.
    A. Stroke volume increases.
    B. Heart rate decreases.
        1. Heart has longer to rest.
        2. Heart has longer to fill with blood.
        3. Heart has longer to receive its own source of oxygen.
    C. Cardiac output increases.

II. Circulatory system becomes more efficient.
    A. Size of blood vessels increases.
    B. Number of blood vessels increases.
    C. Tone of blood vessels increases.
    D. Arterial blood pressure decreases.
    E. Efficiency of myocardial blood distribution increases.
    F. Efficiency of peripheral blood distribution increases.

III. Blood becomes a better transporter.
    A. Number of red blood cells increases.
    B. Mass of red blood cells increases.
    C. Amount of hemoglobin increases.
    D. Amount of plasma increases.
    E. Total blood volume increases (about one quart in average male).
    F. Platelet stickiness decreases.
    G. Levels of triglycerides and cholesterols decrease.
    H. Electron transport capacity increases.
    I. Arterial oxygen content increases.

IV. Other beneficial adaptations.
    A. Glucose intolerance decreases.
    B. Obesity/adiposity decreases.
    C. Thyroid function increases.
    D. Growth hormone production increases.
    E. Vulnerability to dysrhythmias decreases.
    F. Maximal oxygen uptake increases.
    G. Endurance of respiratory muscles increases.
    H. Endurance of locomotor muscles increases.

V. Other possible adaptations.
   A. Improved sleep.
   B. Improved digestion.
   C. Improved elimination.
   D. Improved tolerance to stress.
   E. Improved self-confidence/esteem.
   F. Improved "joie de vivre" including mental and emotional health.

Source: Fox, Samuel M., Naughton, John P., and Gormon, Patrick A. Physical activity and cardiovascular health. *Modern Concepts of Cardiovascular Health* 41(April, 1972):20.

Appendix D

Strength Training Checklist

The following guidelines are basic to a safe, enjoyable, and effective program of strength development. Review your personal training approach in terms of this checklist.

1. Wear a minimum amount of clothing (i.e., T-shirt, shorts).
2. Wear well-made, supportive athletic shoes.
3. Provide ample space to ensure freedom of movement while performing weightlifting exercises.
4. Engage in a few minutes of warm-up activity (e.g., cycling, rope jumping) before beginning the weight workout.
5. Perform static stretching exercises appropriate for each of the muscle groups that will be stressed during the training session.
6. Lift and lower the weights with a moderate and controlled rhythm.
7. Keep the weights evenly balanced throughout the lifting movements.
8. Inhale and exhale with each repetition. Do not hold your breath when lifting weights.
9. Postpone your scheduled workout if the muscles are still fatigued and recuperating from the previous training session.
10. Attempt to maintain regular training days, but do not train when you are not feeling well (e.g., chest cold).
11. Maintain a weight training notebook for reference and motivational purposes.
12. Whenever possible, train with a partner for safety and encouragement.

13. Try not to compare yourself with others. Remember that each person develops muscular strength at a different rate due to inherent physiological and biomechanical factors.

14. Incorporate jogging, swimming, cycling, or some other endurance type activity into your overall training program. Such activities strengthen the heart and improve the function of the circulatory system to help meet the demands of larger, more active muscles.

15. Performing a few minutes of easy, large muscle activity (e.g., walking, jogging, swimming) after a strenuous weight training workout may aid lactic acid removal from the muscles.

16. For optimal training effects, eat a wide variety of nutritious foods (i.e., lean meats, fruits, vegetables, low-fat dairy products, and whole grains) and obtain ample sleep (seven to nine hours nightly).

Appendix E

Strength Training Logbook

Date _____ Start Time _____
Finish Time _____ Workout Time _____

Exercise: _____   Exercise: _____   Exercise: _____
Weightload: _____   Weightload: _____   Weightload: _____
Repetitions: _____   Repetitions: _____   Repetitions: _____
Notes: _____   Notes: _____   Notes: _____

Exercise: _____   Exercise: _____   Exercise: _____
Weightload: _____   Weightload: _____   Weightload: _____
Repetitions: _____   Repetitions: _____   Repetitions: _____
Notes: _____   Notes: _____   Notes: _____

Exercise: _____   Exercise: _____   Exercise: _____
Weightload: _____   Weightload: _____   Weightload: _____
Repetitions: _____   Repetitions: _____   Repetitions: _____
Notes: _____   Notes: _____   Notes: _____

Exercise: _____   Exercise: _____   Exercise: _____
Weightload: _____   Weightload: _____   Weightload: _____
Repetitions: _____   Repetitions: _____   Repetitions: _____
Notes: _____   Notes: _____   Notes: _____

Rest period since last workout: _____
Bodyweight: _____
Measurements: _____

Feelings: Strong   Average   Weak
              Energetic   Average   Tired
              Enthusiastic   Average   Unenthusiastic

Appendix F

YMCA Leg Extension Test for Muscle Strength

EQUIPMENT: Nautilus Leg Extension machine

PERSONNEL: One trained fitness instructor

PROCEDURES:

- Place selector pin in weight stack to lift a resistance that is about 30 percent of your body weight.
- Sit on the Nautilus Leg Extension machine with your knee joints in line with the machine axis of rotation. Place an extra pad behind your back if necessary. Place your ankles behind the roller pad. Fasten the seat belt and place your hands loosely on the handgrips.
- Perform ten slow repetitions in the following manner:

  1. Take two seconds to lift the roller pad to full knee extension.
  2. Hold the fully contracted position for one second.
  3. Take four seconds to lower the roller pad until the weight stack almost touches the support block.

- If you complete ten repetitions, place the selector pin in the weight stack to lift about 40–50 percent of your body weight. After a two-minute rest, perform ten slow repetitions in the same manner as before.

- If you complete ten repetitions, place the selector pin in the weight stack to lift about 60–70 percent of your body weight. After a two-minute rest, perform ten slow repetitions in the same manner as before.
- Continue to test in this manner until you cannot complete ten repetitions in proper form.
- Record the heaviest weight load that you were able to lift ten times with proper form.
- Divide this weight load by your body weight to determine the strength quotient.
- Place your strength quotient in the appropriate strength fitness category.

Strength fitness classifications

Strength quotient	Men	Women
Low	49% and below	39% and below
Below average	50%–59%	40%–49%
Average	60%–69%	50%–59%
Above average	70%–79%	60%–69%
High	80% and above	70% and above

EXAMPLE:

Name:	Jane Smith	Date:	12-06-86
Age:	18	Sex:	Female
Body weight:	100 lbs		

1st weight load:	30 lbs.	for	10 Repetitions
2nd weight load:	50 lbs.	for	10 Repetitions
3rd weight load:	60 lbs.	for	10 Repetitions
4th weight load:	70 lbs.	for	6 Repetitions

Heaviest weight load performed 10 times: 60 lbs.

Divided by body weight: 0.60

Strength quotient: 60%

Strength fitness score: Above average

Source: Westcott, Wayne L. 1986. *Building strength at the YMCA*. Champaign, IL: Human Kinetics Publishing Company.

Appendix G

Strength Training Recommendations for Prepubescent Boys and Girls

In August 1985, the American Orthopaedic Society for Sports Medicine, along with the American Academy of Pediatrics, the American College of Sports Medicine, the National Athletic Trainers Association, the National Strength and Conditioning Association, the President's Council on Physical Fitness and Sports, the Society of Pediatric Orthopaedics, and the U.S. Olympic Committee, developed the following guidelines for prepubescent strength training.

Equipment

1. Strength training equipment should be of appropriate design to accommodate the size and degree of maturity of the prepubescent.
2. It should be cost-effective.
3. It should be safe, free of defects, and inspected frequently.
4. It should be located in an uncrowded area free of obstructions with adequate lighting and ventilation.

Program Considerations

1.   A preparticipation physical exam is mandatory.
2.   The child must have the emotional maturity to accept coaching and instruction.
3.   There must be adequate supervision by coaches who are knowledgeable about strength training and the special problems of prepubescents.
4.   Strength training should be a part of an overall comprehensive program designed to increase motor skills and level of fitness.
5.   Strength training should be preceded by a warm-up period and followed by a cool down.
6.   Emphasis should be on dynamic concentric contractions.
7.   All exercises should be carried through a full range of motion.
8.   Competition is prohibited.
9.   No maximum lift should ever be attempted.

Prescribed Program

1.   Training is recommended two or three times a week for twenty to thirty minute periods.
2.   No resistance should be applied until proper form is demonstrated. Six to fifteen repetitions equal one set; one to three sets per exercise should be done.
3.   Weight or resistance is increased in one to three pound increments after the prepubescent does fifteen repetitions in good form.

Glossary

Abduction: Sideward movement away from the midline of the body.

Activity Time: Time spent in actual training activity (i.e., performing exercises) as differentiated from time spent in a training facility.

Adduction: Sideward movements toward the midline of the body.

Adenosine Triphosphate (ATP):   The chemical compound that, when split, produces the energy for muscular contraction.

Aerobic: Activities that require large amounts of oxygen to produce energy for sustained periods of exercise.

Anaerobic Glycolysis: The breakdown of glycogen in the absence of oxygen to produce energy for vigorous activity lasting between thirty seconds and three minutes.

Antagonistic Muscle: The muscle that produces the opposite joint action to the prime mover muscle.

Assisted Training: A strength training technique characterized by helping the exerciser perform a few additional repetitions after muscle failure has occured with the selected resistance.

Atrophy: Decrease in the cross-sectional size of a muscle.

Berger Program: A system of strength training in which the exerciser performs three sets of six repetitions each. All three sets are done with the 6-RM weightload.

Bodybuilders: Persons who use strength training as a means for achieving a better muscular appearance, especially with regard to muscle size, shape, definition, and proportion.

Body Composition: The relationship between fat tissue and lean body tissue such as muscle, bone, blood, skin, and organs. Recommended body composition for males is less than 15 percent fat. Recommended body composition for females is less than 20 percent fat.

Bodyweight Exercises: Exercises in which one's bodyweight serves as the resistance. Some bodyweight exercises can be augmented by attaching barbell plates to the waist.

Breakdown Training: A strength training technique characterized by immediately reducing the resistance at the point of muscle failure and performing a few additional repetitions to further stress the muscles.

Circuit Training: A training program in which one moves immediately from an exercise for one muscle group (e.g., shoulders) to an exercise for a different muscle group (e.g., abdominals), and so on until each major muscle group has been worked.

Concentric Contraction: A contraction in which a muscle exerts force, shortens, and overcomes a resistance.

Controlled Movement Speed: A weightload is raised and lowered in a slow and controlled manner to provide consistent application of force throughout the exercise movement.

DeLorme-Watkins Program: A system of strength training in which the exerciser performs three sets of ten repetitions each. The first set is done with 50 percent of the 10-RM weightload, the second set is executed with 75 percent of the 10-RM weightload, and the third set is completed with 100 percent of the 10-RM weightload.

Diastolic Blood Pressure: The lowest pressure inside the artery walls associated with the resting phase of the heart (diastole).

Direct Resistance: The resistive force is applied to the same body segment (e.g., upper arm) to which the movement force is applied.

Eccentric Contraction: A contraction in which a muscle exerts force, lengthens, and is overcome by a resistance.

Endurance: A measure of one's ability to continue exercising with a given, submaximum workload.

Extension: A movement that increases the joint angle between adjacent body parts.

Fasiculi: Groups of muscle fibers bound together by a membrane called perimysium.

Fast-Twitch Muscle Fibers: Muscle fibers that possess a greater capacity for anaerobic energy production.

First-Class Lever: Lever arrangement in which the axis of rotation is between the movement force and the resistance.

Flexion: A movement that decreases the joint angle between adjacent body parts.

Free Weights: Barbells and dumbbells are usually referred to as free weights or loose weights because there are no restrictions on how they are utilized.

Full-Range Movement: Exercising a muscle through a complete range of joint motion, from a position of full extension to a position of full flexion, and vice versa.

Fusiform: Muscles characterized by relatively long fibers that run parallel to the line of pull.

High-Endurance Muscles: Muscles with a large percentage of slow-twitch fibers that tend to fatigue slowly.

Hypertrophy: Increase in the cross-sectional size of a muscle.

Isokinetic Training: Training on apparatus that automatically varies the resistance in accordance with the applied muscle force. In isokinetic exercise, the amount of muscle force produced determines the amount of resistive force encountered.

Isometric Contraction: A contraction in which a muscle exerts force but does not change in length.

Isometric Training: Strength training that involves static (isometric) contractions. In isometric exercise there is muscle tension but no muscle movement.

Isotonic Training: Strength training that involves positive and negative contractions. In isotonic exercise the amount of resistive force selected determines the amount of muscle force required.

Keiser Equipment: One type of isotonic exercise machine that provides variable resistance by means of air pressure.

Lactic Acid: A fatigue-producing by-product of anaerobic glycolysis.

Low-Endurance Muscles: Muscles with a large percentage of fast-twitch fibers that tend to fatigue quickly.

Maximum Heart Rate The fastest rate that one's heart will contract. Maximum heart rate can be estimated by subtracting one's age from 220. For example, a typical forty-year old man or woman would have a maximum heart rate of 180 beats per minute ($220 - 40 = 180$ beats per minute).

Maximum Oxygen Uptake: Often referred to as Max V02, this represents the greatest amount of oxygen one can utilize during high levels of endurance exercise.

Motor Unit: A single motor neuron and all the muscle fibers that receive stimulation from that nerve.

Multi-joint Exercise: Exercise that involves two or more joint actions and two or more major muscle groups. Linear movements such as bench presses, dips, chins and squats are multi-joint exercises.

Muscle Balance: Maintaining a natural strength ratio between opposing muscle groups and training for overall muscular development, rather than specializing on particular muscles or exercises.

Muscle Belly: The actual muscle length between the tendon attachments.

Muscle Density: The relationship of muscle tissue and fat tissue within a muscle area. Low-density muscle areas contain large amounts of fat. High-density muscle areas contain small amounts of fat. High-density muscles are stronger, firmer, and have higher energy requirements.

Muscle Failure: The point during an exercise set when the muscle is no longer able to contract concentrically and is temporarily overcome by the resistance.

Muscle Fibers: Groups of myofibrils bound together by a membrane called sarcolema, and innervated by a motor neuron.

Muscle Isolation: Designing training exercises so that the movement is accomplished to as large a degree as possible by a single muscle group, such as the Nautilus Multi-Triceps Machine to focus on the triceps muscles.

Muscle Pump: High-intensity training that saturates the target muscle tissue with blood and temporarily increases the cross-sectional area. This process is often referred to as "pumping-up" the muscles.

Myofibrils: The principal threads running throughout the muscles, myofibrils are formed from adjacent sarcomeres.

Nautilus Equipment: One type of isotonic exercise equipment, most Nautilus machines provide supportive structure, direct resistance, rotary movement, and automatically variable resistance, which appear to enhance muscle isolation and stress intensification.

Near-Maximum Resistance: Weightloads exceeding 65 percent of maximum are most effective for developing muscle strength and are referred to as near-maximum resistance.

Negative Training: A strength training technique characterized by emphasizing the negative (eccentric) phase of exercise to develop greater muscle tension.

Olympic Lifters: Persons who train with weights in order to lift heavier weightloads in their competitive events, the clean and jerk and the snatch.

One Repetition Maximum (1 RM):   The heaviest weightload a person can lift once is called the one repetition maximum (1 RM) weightload.

Overload: Using progressively more resistance than the muscles are accustomed to in order to stimulate positive strength adaptations. Overload is a relative term as a true overload would not permit concentric muscle contractions.

Overtraining: Exercising so hard that the muscles do not fully recover and rebuild between training sessions resulting in strength decrement rather than strength increment.

Paired Exercises: Following an exercise for a given muscle group with an exercise for the antagonistic muscle group. For example, performing leg curls (hamstrings) upon completing leg extensions (quadriceps).

Penniform: Muscles characterized by relatively short fibers that run diagonally to the line of pull.

Phosphagen: The primary source of energy for vigorous activity of a few seconds' duration.

Postpubertal: Postpubertal refers to young men and women who have reached sexual maturity, or puberty.

Power: Power is defined as the rate at which work is performed. Technically, power is the product of muscle force and movement speed, which means that power can be enhanced by increasing muscle force, movement speed, or both.

Powerlifters: Persons who train with weights in order to lift heavier weightloads in their competitive events, the squat, dead lift, and bench press.

Prepubertal: Prepubertal refers to children who have not reached sexual maturity, or puberty.

Prestretching: A quick stretching (lengthening) of a muscle just prior to contraction that enables the muscle to produce greater force.

Prime Mover Muscle: In any given joint action, the muscle that contracts concentrically to accomplish the movement.

Pyramid Program: A system of strength training in which the exerciser performs successive sets utilizing increasing weightloads and decreasing repetitions. One type of pyramid program consists of ten repetitions with 55 percent of the 1-RM weightload, five repetitions with 75 percent of the 1-RM weightload, and one repetition with 95 percent of the 1-RM weightload.

Rebuilding Time: The time required for the muscles to rebuild to a higher level of strength following a training session.

Reciprocal Inhibition: The nervous regulatory process that enables an antagonist muscle to relax and lengthen when a prime mover muscle contracts and shortens.

Recovery Time: The rest time allowed for the muscles to partially recover between successive sets of exercise.

Repetitions: The number of times an exercise is performed in succession. For example, the exerciser who takes the barbell from the floor, presses it ten times, and returns it to the floor has completed one set of ten repetitions.

Repetition Maximum: Refers to the maximum resistance one can use for a given number of repetitions. For example, one's five-repetition maximum is the heaviest weightload that can be performed for five repetitions.

Rotary Movement: Movement in a circular pathway, ideally with the resistance axis of rotation in line with the joint axis of rotation.

Sarcomere: The smallest functional unit of muscle contraction, a sarcomere consists of thin actin filaments, thick myosin filaments, and tiny cross-bridges that serve as coupling agents between these two protein structures.

Second-Class Lever: Lever arrangement in which the resistance is between the axis of rotation and the movement force.

Set: The number of separate exercise bouts performed. For example, the exerciser who does ten bench presses, rests a minute, then does ten more bench presses has completed two sets of ten repetitions each.

Slow-Twitch Muscle Fibers: Muscle fibers that have a greater capacity for aerobic energy production.

Spotter: A training partner who gives assistance with an unsuccessful lifting attempt, adds resistance during an exercise, provides encouragement and feedback, and otherwise helps the exerciser train in a safe and effective manner. Spotters should be present in exercises such as the bench press and squat for safety reasons.

Stabilizer Muscle: A muscle that stabilizes one joint so that the desired movement can be performed in another joint.

Strength: A measure of one's ability to exert muscular force against a resistance.

Strength Plateau: A period of time during which no further strength gains occur. It indicates that some aspect of the training program should be changed to enable further progress.

Strength Quotient: A means of comparing muscle strength among individuals of different sizes. The strength quotient is determined by dividing the maximum weight lifted in a given exercise by the exerciser's bodyweight. For example, a 150 pound person who can bench press a maximum weightload of 300 pounds has a strength quotient of 2.0.

Stress Adaptation: The ability of a muscle to respond positively to progressively greater training demands by gradually increasing contractile strength.

Stress Intensification: Progressively increasing the contractile demands of the muscles by training with more resistance, more repetitions, slower movements, or other means for making the exercise more difficult.

Stretch Reflex: When a muscle is suddenly stretched, specialized control mechanisms called muscle spindles automatically trigger a rapid and forceful muscle contraction known as the stretch reflex or myotatic reflex.

Super-Slow Training: A strength training technique characterized by very slow (ten second) lifting movements to reduce the role of momentum and increase muscle tension.

Systolic Blood Pressure: The highest pressure inside the artery walls associated with the pumping phase of the heart (systole).

Ten Repetition Maximum (10-RM): The heaviest weightload an exerciser can lift ten times in succession is referred to as the 10-RM weightload. Most people can perform ten repetitions with about 75 percent of their maximum weightload.

Third-Class Lever: Lever arrangement in which the movement force is applied between the axis of rotation and the resistance.

Training Duration: The duration of a training set is the time from the first to the last repetition. The duration of a training session is the time from the beginning to the end of the workout.

Training Intensity: The degree of effort involved in an exercise set. Generally speaking, high intensity strength training requires sixty to ninety seconds of very hard effort resulting in muscle failure.

Training Principles: Research based guidelines for developing muscle strength in a safe and effective manner.

Training Specificity: Training in a specific manner to achieve specific objectives. For example, leg extensions with a 10-RM weightload would be more effective for strengthening the quadriceps muscles than a ten-mile run.

Training Volume: Training volume is the total amount of work performed (weight lifted) during a training session. This can be calculated by multiplying each exercise weightload by the number of repetitions performed and summing the totals.

Universal Gym: One type of isotonic exercise machine that provides a variety of exercise stations at which smooth running weight-stacks are lifted by lever and pulley attachments.

Valsalva Response: Holding the breath during a strenuous lifting movement produces increased pressure in the chest area, which can interfere with venous blood return to the heart and significantly elevate blood pressure.

Variable Resistance Training: Training on an apparatus that automatically changes the resistance throughout the exercise range of movement to accommodate the variations in muscle strength at different joint angles.

Work: The amount of work performed is the product of the force (weightload) multiplied by the distance traveled.

Bibliography

American College of Sports Medicine. 1980. *Guidelines for graded exercise testing and exercise prescription.* Philadelphia: Lea and Febiger.

Astrand, Per-Olof, and Rodahl, Kaare. 1977. *Textbook of work physiology, second edition.* New York: McGraw-Hill.

Atherton, G. W., James, N. T., and Mahan, M. 1981. Studies on muscle fibre splitting in skeletal muscle. *Experientia,* 37:308–310.

Baratta, R., Solomonow, M., et al. 1988. Muscular coactivation. *American Journal of Sports Medicine,* 16:113–122.

Berger, Richard A. 1962a. Effects of varied weight training programs on strength. *Research Quarterly,* 33:168–181.

Berger, Richard A. 1962b. Optimum repetitions for the development of strength. *Research Quarterly,* 33:334–338.

Berger, Richard A. 1963. Comparative effects of three weight training programs. *Research Quarterly,* 34:396–397.

Berger, Richard A. 1965. Comparison of the effects of various weight training loads on strength. *Research Quarterly,* 36:141–146.

Byrnes, William C., and Clarkson, Priscilla M. 1986. Delayed onset muscle soreness and training. *Clinics in Sports Medicine,* 5:605–614 (July).

Cahill, B. R., and Griffith, E. H. 1978. Effects of pre-season conditioning on the incidence and severity of high school football knee injuries. *American Journal of Sports Medicine,* 6:180–183.

Clark, Nancy. 1985. Calorie adaptations to exercise. *Boston Running News,* 3:14–15.

Clarke, David H., and Manning, James M. 1985. Properties of isokinetic fatigue at various movement speeds in adult males. *Research Quarterly for Exercise and Sport,* 56:221–226.

Clarke, H. Harrison. 1971. *Physical and motor tests in the Medford boys' growth study*. Englewood Cliffs, N.J.: Prentice-Hall.

Clarkson, Priscilla. 1984. Muscle physiology and muscle fatigue. Paper presented at Northeast Region YMCA Strength Fitness Seminar, Greenfield, Massachusetts, September 30.

Costill, D. L., Coyle, E. F., Fink, W. F., Lesmes, G. R., and Witzmann, F. A. 1979. Adaptations in skeletal muscle following strength training. *Journal of Applied Physiology*, 46:96–99.

Counsilman, J. 1976. The importance of speed in exercise. *Scholastic Coach*, 46:94–99.

Coyle, E. F., Feiring, D. C., Rotkis, T. C., et al. 1981. Specificity of power improvements through slow and fast isokinetic training. *Journal of Applied Physiology*, 51:1437–1442.

Darden, Ellington. 1977. *Strength training principles: How to get the most out of your workouts*. Winter Park, Fla.: Anna Publishing Company, Inc.

Darden, Ellington, 1981. *The Nautilus nutrition book*. Chicago: Contemporary Books, Inc.

Darden, Ellington, 1988. *The Nautilus book*. Chicago: Contemporary Books, Inc.

DeLorme, Thomas L., and Watkins, Arthur L. 1948. Techniques of progressive resistance exercise. *Archives of Physical Medicine*, 29:263.

Dons, B., Bollerup, K., Bonde-Peterson, F., and Hancke, S. 1979. The effect of weight lifting exercise related to muscle fiber composition and muscle cross-sectional area in humans. *European Journal of Applied Physiology*, 40:95–106.

Duda, Marty. 1986. Prepubescent strength training gains support. *Physician and Sportsmedicine*, 14:157–161.

Evans, William J. 1987. Exercise-induced skeletal muscle damage. *Physician and Sportsmedicine*, 15:89–100.

Finamore, Leonard V. 1989. Survey of Massachusetts high school football team strength and conditioning programs. Master's thesis. Vermont College of Norwich University.

Fleck, S. J., and Falkel, J. E. 1986. Value of resistance training for the reduction of sports injuries. *Sports Medicine*, 3:61–68.

Fleck, S. J., and Kraemer, W. J. 1987. *Designing resistance training programs*. Champaign, Ill.: Human Kinetics Publishing Company.

Forbes, G. B. 1976. The adult decline in lean body mass. *Human Biology*, 48:161–173.

Fox, Edward L. 1979. *Sports physiology*. Philadelphia: W. B. Saunders.

Freedson, P., Chang, B., and Katch, F. 1984. Intra-arterial blood pressure during free-weight and hydraulic resistive exercise. *Medicine and Science in Sports and Exercise,* 16:131.

Friden, J., Sjostrom, M., and Ekblom, B. 1983. Myofibrillar damage following intense eccentric exercise in man. *International Journal of Sports Medicine,* 3:170–176.

Fukunaga, T. 1976. Die absolute muskelkraft und das muskelkrafttraining. *Sportarzt und Sportmed,* 11:255–265. As reported in McDonagh, M. J. N., and Davies, C. T. M. 1984. Adaptive response of mammalian skeletal muscle to exercise with high loads. *European Journal of Applied Physiology,* 52:139–155.

Gettman, L. R., and Ayres, J. 1978. Aerobic changes through 10 weeks of slow and fast isokinetic training (abstract). *Medicine and Science in Sports,* 10:47.

Goldberg, L. E., Schutz, R., and Kloster, F. 1983. Improvement in cardiovascular response to exercise after weight training. *Clinical Research,* 31:9.

Goldberg, L., Elliot, D. L., Schultz, R. W., and Kloster, F. E. 1984. Changes in lipid and lipoprotein levels after weight training. *Journal of the American Medical Association,* 252:504–506.

Golding, Lawrence A., Meyers, Clayton R., and Sinning, Wayne E. 1982. *The Y's way to physical fitness.* Chicago: YMCA of the USA.

Gordon, H. H. 1967. Anatomical and biomechanical adaptations of muscles to different exercises. *Journal of the American Medical Association,* 201:755–758.

Hagberg, J. M., Eksani, A. A., Goldring, O., et al. 1984. Effect of weight training on blood pressure and hemodynamics in hypertensive adolescents. *Journal of Pediatrics,* 104:147–151.

Hakkinen, K., and Komi, P. 1983. Electromyographic changes during strength training and detraining. *Medicine and Science in Sports and Exercise,* 15:455–460.

Harris, Kathryn A., and Holly, Robert G. 1987. Physiological response to circuit weight training in borderline hypertensive subjects. *Medicine and Science in Sports and Exercise,* 19:246–252.

Hejna, W. F., Buturusis, W., Rosenberg, A., et al. 1982. Prevention of sports injuries in high school students through strength training. *National Strength and Conditioning Association Journal,* 4:28–31.

Hempel, Linda S., and Wells, Christine L. 1985. Cardiorespiratory cost of the Nautilus express circuit. *The Physician and Sportsmedicine,* 13:82–97.

Hettinger, Theodore. 1961. *Physiology of strength.* Springfield, Ill.: Charles C. Thomas.

Hunter, G. R., and McCarthy, J. P. 1982. Pressure response associated with high-intensity anaerobic training. *The Physician and Sportsmedicine*, 11:151–162.

Hurley, B. F., Hagberg, J. M., Goldberg, A. P., et al. 1988. Resistive training can reduce coronary risk factors without altering VO2 max or percent body fat. *Medicine and Science in Sports and Exercise*, 20:150–154.

Hurley, B. F., Seals, D. R., Ehsani, A. A., Cartier, L. J., Dalsky, G. P., Hagberg, J. M., and Holloszy, J. O. 1984. Effects of high-intensity strength training on cardiovascular function. *Medicine and Science in Sports and Exercise*, 16:483–488.

Huxley, H. 1969. The mechanism of muscular contraction. *Science*, 164:1356–1366.

Ikai, M., and Fukunaga, T. 1970. A study on training effect on strength per unit cross-sectional area of muscle by means of ultrasonic measurement. *European Journal of Applied Physiology*, 28:173–180.

Ikai, M., and Steinhaus, A. H. 1961. Some factors modifying the expression of human strength. *Journal of Applied Physiology*, 16:157–163.

Johnson, C. C., Stone, M. H., Lopez, A., Hebert, J. A., and Kilgore, I. T. 1982. Diet and exercise in middle-aged men. *Journal of the American Dietetic Association*, 81:695–701.

Johnson, LaVon. 1986. The role of muscle in high-level wellness. *The Winning Edge*, 5:1, 5, 12 (March–April).

Jones, A., Pollock, M., Graves, J., et al. 1988. *Safe, specific testing and rehabilitative exercise for the muscles of the lumbar spine.* Santa Barbara, Calif.: Sequoia Communications.

Jones, Arthur. 1986. Exercise 1986: The present state of the art; now a science. *Club Industry*, 2:36A–64A.

Karpovich, Peter V., and Sinning, Wayne E. 1971. *Physiology of muscular activity.* Philadelphia: W. B. Saunders.

Katch, Frank I., and Drumm, Sarah S. 1986. Effects of different modes of strength training on body composition and anthropometry. *Clinics in Sports Medicine*, 5:413–459 (July).

Kelemen, Michael H., Stewart, Kerry J., Gillilan, Ronald E., et al. 1986. Circuit weight training in cardiac patients. *Journal of the American College of Cardiology*, 7:38–42 (January).

Keyes, A., Taylor, H. L., and Grande, F. 1973. Basal metabolism and age of adult man. *Metabolism*, 22:579–587.

Lamb, David R. 1978. *Physiology of exercise: Responses and adaptations.* New York: Macmillan.

Lamb, Lawrence E. 1985. Understanding calorie use and loss. *The Health Letter*, 27:1–4 (February).

Legwold, Gary. 1982. Does lifting weights harm a prepubescent athlete? *Physician and Sportsmedicine*, 10:141–144.

Lesmes, George R., Benham, David W., Costill, David L., and Fink, William J. 1983. Glycogen utilization in fast- and slow-twitch muscle fibers during maximal isokinetic exercise. *Annals of Sports Medicine*, 1:105–108.

MacDougall, J. D., 1985a. Determining factors of strength: Part one. *National Strength and Conditioning Association Journal*, 7:10–23 (February–March).

MacDougall, J. D. 1985b. Determining factors of strength: Part two. *National Strength and Conditioning Association Journal*, 7:10–17 (April–May).

MacDougall, J. D., Sale, D. G., Elden, G. C. B., and Sutton, J. R. 1982. Muscle ultrastructural characteristics of elite powerlifters and body-builders. *European Journal of Applied Physiology*, 48:117–126.

MacDougall, J. D., Tuxen, D., Sale, D., Sexton, A., Moroz, J., and Sutton, J., 1983. Direct measurement of arterial blood pressure during heavy resistance training. *Medicine and Science in Sports and Exercise*, 15:158.

Mathews, Donald K., and Fox, Edward L. 1976. *The physiological basis of physical education and athletics*. Philadelphia: W. B. Saunders.

McDonagh, M. J., and Davies, C. T. 1984. Adaptive response of mammalian skeletal muscles to exercise with high loads. *European Journal of Applied Physiology*, 52:139–155.

Melleby, Alexander. 1982. *The Y's way to a healthy back*. Piscataway, N.J.: New Century.

Messier, Stephen P., and Dill, Mary. 1985. Alterations in strength and maximal oxygen uptake consequent to Nautilus circuit weight training. *Research Quarterly for Exercise and Sport*, 56:345–351.

Micheli, L. 1983. Preadolescents show dramatic strength gains. *The Physician and Sportsmedicine*, 11:25.

Micheli, Lyle J. 1985. Physiological and orthopedic considerations for strengthening the prepubescent athlete. *National Strength and Conditioning Association Journal*, 7:26–27.

Misner, J. E., Boileau, R. A., Massey, B. H., and Mayhew, J. L. 1974. Alterations in the body composition of adult men during selected physical training programs. *Journal of the American Geriatric Society*, 22:33–38.

Moffroid, Mary T., and Whipple, Robert H. 1970. Specificity of speed and exercise. *Journal of the American Physical Therapy Association*, 50:1692–1699.

Morganroth, J., Maron, B., Henry, W., and Epstein, S. 1975. Comparative left ventricular dimensions in trained athletes. *Annals of International Medicine*, 82:521–524.

Moritani, T., and DeVries, H. 1979. Neural factors versus hypertrophy in the time course of muscle strength gain. *American Journal of Physical Medicine*, 58:115-130.

Mueller, F. O., and Blyth, C. S. 1982. Fatalities and catastrophic injuries in football. *The Physician and Sportsmedicine*, 10:135-138.

Myers, Clayton R. 1975. *The official YMCA physical fitness handbook*. New York: Popular Library.

Nutter, J. 1986. Physical activity increases bone density. *National Strength and Conditioning Association Journal*, 8:67-69.

O'Shea, Patrick. 1966. Effects of selected weight training programs on the development of muscle hypertrophy. *Research Quarterly*, 37:95.

Palmieri, Gerard A. 1987. Weight training and repetition speed. *Journal of Applied Sport Science Research*, 1:36-38.

Peterson, James. 1982. *Total fitness: the Nautilus way*. West Point, N. Y.: Leisure Press.

Peterson, James A. 1976. The effect of high-intensity weight training on cardiovascular function. Paper presented at International Congress of Physical Activity Sciences, Quebec City, July 15.

Pipes, T. V. 1978. Variable resistance versus constant resistance strength training in adult males. *European Journal of Applied Physiology*, 39:27-35.

Pipes, T. V. 1979. High intensity, not high speed. *Athletic Journal*, 59:60-62.

Pipes, T. V., and Wilmore, J. H. 1975. Isokinetic vs. isotonic strength training in adult men. *Medicine and Science in Sports and Exercise*, 7:262-274.

Pollock, Michael L., Wilmore, Jack H., and Fox, Samuel M. 1978. *Health and fitness through physical activity*. New York: John Wiley and Sons.

President's Council on Physical Fitness and Sports. 1985. *National school population fitness survey*. HHS—Office of the Assistant Secretary for Health, Washington, D.C.

Rhoades, Dale, and Westcott, Wayne L. 1986. Relationship between repetitions and weightloads in bench press and squat. *American Fitness Quarterly*, 6:7, 26.

Ricci, G., Lajoie, D., and Petitelerc, R. 1982. Left ventricular size following endurance, sprint, and strength training. *Medicine and Science in Sports and Exercise*, 14:344-347.

Riley, Daniel B. 1982. *Strength training: by the experts*. West Point, N. Y.: Leisure Press.

Schantz, P. 1982. Capillary supply in hypertrophied human skeletal muscle. *Acta Physiologica Scandinavia*, 114:635-637.

Sewall, Les, and Micheli, Lyle J. 1986. Strength training for children. *Journal of Pediatric Orthopedics*, 6:143–146.

Siegel, Judy. 1988. Fitness in prepubescent children: Implications for exercise training. *National Strength and Conditioning Association Journal*, 10:43–48.

Stone, M. H., Blessing, D., Byrd, R., Tew, J., and Boatwright, D. 1982. Physiological effects of a short term resistive training program on middle-aged untrained men. *National Strength and Conditioning Association Journal*, 4:16–20.

Stone, Michael H., Wilson, G. D., and Blessing, D. 1983. Cardiovascular responses to short-term Olympic style weight training in young men. *Canadian Journal of Applied Sport Science*, 8:134–139.

Stone, William J., and Kroll, William A. 1978. *Sports conditioning and weight training*. Boston: Allyn and Bacon.

Vander, Lauren B., Franklin, Barry A., Wrisley, David, and Rubenfire, Melvyn. 1986. Acute cardiovascular responses to Nautilus exercise in cardiac patients: Implications for exercise training. *Annals of Sports Medicine*, 2:165–169.

Ward, Ann. 1988. Time course of physiologic changes during interval and steady state cycle training. Paper presented at American College of Sports Medicine Annual Meeting, Dallas, Texas, May 1988.

Weltman, Arthur, Janney, Carol, Rians, Clark B., et al. 1986. The effects of hydraulic resistance strength training in pre-pubertal males. *Medicine and Science in Sports and Exercise*, 18:629–638.

Westcott, Wayne L. 1974. Effects of varied frequencies of weight training on the development of strength. Master's thesis. The Pennsylvania State University.

Westcott, Wayne L. 1976. Unpublished research study.

Westcott, Wayne L. 1979a. Female response to weight training. *Journal of Physical Education*, 77:31–33.

Westcott, Wayne L. 1979b. Physical educators and coaches as models of behavior. *Journal of Physical Education and Recreation*, 50:31–32 (March).

Westcott, Wayne L. 1980. Effects of teacher modeling on children's peer encouragement behavior. *Research Quarterly for Exercise and Sport*, 51:585–587.

Westcott, Wayne L. 1984a. Effects of strength training on women studied by YMCA. *Journal of Physical Education and Program*, 81:H8–H9 (December).

Westcott, Wayne L. 1984b. The case for slow weight training technique. *Scholastic Coach*, 54:42–44 (August).

Westcott, Wayne L. 1984c. Modern currents in weight training. *Scholastic Coach*, 54:53 (November).

Westcott, Wayne L. 1985a. The inevitable strength plateau. *Scholastic Coach*, 55:30–31 (September).

Westcott, Wayne L. 1985b. Cardiovascular fitness and strength training. Paper presented at Nautilus National Fitness Seminar, Las Vegas, August 8, 1985.

Westcott, Wayne L. 1985c. Combating disappointment when strength training progress slows. *The Journal of Physical Education and Program*, 81:D14–D15 (June).

Westcott, Wayne L. 1985d. Weight loss and weight gain. *Scholastic Coach*, 55:16–17 (December).

Westcott, Wayne L. 1985e. What happens when the athlete misses a strength workout? *Scholastic Coach*, 54:56–57 (March).

Westcott, Wayne L. 1985f. Determining factors of strength: Part one. *National Strength and Conditioning Association Journal*, 7:10–23 (February–March).

Westcott, Wayne L. 1985g. Determining factors of strength: Part two. *National Strength and Conditioning Association Journal*, 7:10–17 (April–May).

Westcott, Wayne L. 1985h. Instructor training: key to Y fitness leadership. *Journal of Physical Education and Program*, 81:F4–F5 (September).

Westcott, Wayne L. 1985i. Provide steak not sizzle with sophisticated technology. *Journal of Physical Education and Program*, 81:G5–G6 (October).

Westcott, Wayne L. 1985j. Bar dips: the one exercise. *Scholastic Coach*, 54:24 (May–June).

Westcott, Wayne L. 1985k. Power: the critical factor. *Scholastic Coach*, 55:52–53 (August).

Westcott, Wayne L. 1985l. The eight basic principles of muscle strengthening. *Scholastic Coach*, 55:22 (November).

Westcott, Wayne L. 1985m. Weight loss and weight gain. *Scholastic Coach*, 5:16–17 (December).

Westcott, Wayne L. 1986a. Muscle development, safety make case for slow strength training. *Journal of Physical Education and Program*, 82:E14–E16 (April).

Westcott, Wayne L. 1986b. Strength training and blood pressure. *American Fitness Quarterly*, 5:38–39.

Westcott, Wayne L. 1986c. New incentives: Weight loss and strength training. *Club Industry*, 2:62–63 (June).

Westcott, Wayne L. 1986d. Losing weight with and without strength training. Paper presented at National YMCA Strength Training Instructor Certification Workshop, San Francisco, Calif., May 1, 1986.

Westcott, Wayne L. 1986e. Comparative effects of two and three strength training sessions per week. Paper presented at National YMCA Strength Instructor Certification Workshop, San Francisco, Calif., May 1, 1986.

Westcott, Wayne L. 1986f. The key to a successful weight training program is instructors who care. *Club Industry*, 2:58–59 (July).

Westcott, Wayne L. 1986g. Integration of strength, endurance, and skill training. *Scholastic Coach*, 55:74 (May–June).

Westcott, Wayne L. 1986h. Comparison of eight repetition training and twelve repetition training with track and field athletes. Paper presented at National YMCA Strength Instructor Certification Workshop, Boston, Mass., April 3, 1986.

Westcott, Wayne L. 1986i. *Building strength at the YMCA*. Champaign, Ill.: Human Kinetics Publishing Company.

Westcott, Wayne L. 1986j. Four key factors in building a strength program. *Scholastic Coach*, 55:104–105 (January).

Westcott, Wayne L. 1986k. Strength training for injury prevention. *Scholastic Coach*, 56:62, 65 (October).

Westcott, Wayne L. 1986l. How many reps per set? *Scholastic Coach*, 56:72–73 (December).

Westcott, Wayne L. 1986m. Good training, communication cited as keys in fitness instructors. *Perspective*, 13:37–40 (October).

Westcott, Wayne L. 1987a. Circuit strength training, an in-season alternative. *Scholastic Coach*, 56:120–121 (January).

Westcott, Wayne L. 1987b. Exercise sessions can make the difference in weight loss. *Perspective*, 13:42–44 (February).

Westcott, Wayne L. 1987c. Motivation crucial to continued growth of strength training. *Perspective*, 13:30–31 (June).

Westcott, Wayne L. 1987d. Individualized strength training for girl high school runners. *Scholastic Coach*, 51:71–72 (December).

Westcott, Wayne L. 1988a. Can you get bigger on Nautilus? *American Fitness Quarterly*, 6:15–16 (January).

Westcott, Wayne L. 1988b. Rethinking your fitness center. *Club Industry*, 4:29–33 (March).

Westcott, Wayne, L. 1988c. Training and testing specificity. *Scholastic Coach*, 57:14, 82 (March).

Westcott, Wayne L. 1988d. Study shows average youth has high percent of body fat. *Perspective*, 14:28–29 (April).

Westcott, Wayne L. 1988e. Now for the good news: Kids can improve body composition. *Perspective*, 14:54–55 (June).

Westcott, Wayne L. 1988f. Strength training. *Sport Care and fitness*, 1:59–62 (July/August).

Westcott, Wayne L. 1988g. Some thoughts about fitness testing. *American Fitness Quarterly*, 7:37, 39 (July).

Westcott, Wayne L. 1988h. Sensible weight training. *IDEA Today*, 6:30–36 (September).

Westcott, Wayne L. 1988i. Four ways for fitness instructors to become good role models. *Perspective*, 14:36–37 (September).

Westcott, Wayne L. 1988j. Fitness testing in the YMCA. Paper presented at the Consensus Meeting of the United States Public Health Service, Washington, D. C., February.

Westcott, Wayne L. 1988k. Unpublished research study.

Westcott, Wayne L. 1988l. Eliminating myths: Does strength training harm blood pressure? *Perspective*, 14:37–39 (December).

Westcott, Wayne L. 1989a. A model for orienting your strength training participants. *Perspective*, 15:28, 30 (January).

Westcott, Wayne L. 1989b. Mighty mites. *SportCare & Fitness*, 2:28–30 (March/April).

Westcott, Wayne L., Benkis, John F., and McPhee, Joseph. 1985. Fitness Evaluation Software. South Shore YMCA, Quincy, Mass.

Westcott, Wayne L., Greenberger, K., and Milius, D. 1989. Strength training research: Sets and repetitions. *Scholastic Coach*, 58:98–100.

Westcott, Wayne L., and Howes, Bernard. 1983. Blood pressure response during weight training exercise. *National Strength and Conditioning Association Journal*, 5:67–71 (February–March).

Westcott, Wayne L., and Pappas, Marilyn. 1987. Immediate effects of circuit strength training on blood pressure. *American Fitness Quarterly*, 6:43–44 (October).

Westcott, Wayne L., and Warren, Thomas G. 1985. Short rest Nautilus training can improve cardiovascular performance. *Journal of Physical Education and Program*, 81:E18–E19 (July).

Wilmore, J. H. 1974. Alterations in strength, body composition and anthropometric measurements consequent to 10-week weight training program. *Medicine and Science in Sports and Exercise*, 6:133–138.

Wilmore, J. H., Parr, R. B., and Ward, P. 1978. Energy cost of circuit weight training. *Medicine and Science in Sports and Exercise*, 10:75–78.

Withers, R. T. 1970. Effects of varied weight training loads on the strength of university freshmen. *Research Quarterly*, 41:110–114.

Wolf, Michael D. 1981. *Muscle: structure, function and control.* Deland, Fl: Nautilus Sports Medical Industries.

Wright, James E. 1978. *Anabolic steroids and sports.* Natick, Mass.: Sports-Science Consultants.

Zohman, Lenore R. 1974. *Exercise your way to fitness and heart health.* Englewood Cliffs, N. J.: CPC International.

Zuckerman, J., and Stull, G. A. 1969. Effects of exercise on knee ligament separation force in rats. *Journal of Applied Physiology,* 26:716–719.

Index

2511